live your life

live your life

MY STORY OF LOVING AND LOSING NICK CORDERO

Amanda Kloots

with Anna Kloots

HARPER

An Imprint of HarperCollins*Publishers*

LIVE YOUR LIFE. Copyright © 2021 by Amanda Kloots. All rights reserved. Printed in the United States of America. No part of this book may be used or reproduced in any manner whatsoever without written permission except in the case of brief quotations embodied in critical articles and reviews. For information, address HarperCollins Publishers, 195 Broadway, New York, NY 10007.

HarperCollins books may be purchased for educational, business, or sales promotional use. For information, please email the Special Markets Department at SPsales@harpercollins.com.

All photos courtesy of the author unless otherwise noted.

FIRST EDITION

Designed by Kyle O'Brien

Library of Congress Cataloging-in-Publication Data has been applied for.

ISBN 978-0-06-307825-3

21 22 23 24 25   LSC   10 9 8 7 6 5 4 3 2 1

For Nick,
Now you know your story

For Elvis,
Now you have his story

prologue

I walked so fast I was almost running down a long, linoleum hallway in Cedars-Sinai Medical Center.

It was 12:13 in the afternoon but looked like two in the morning—the vast atrium was abandoned, with empty chairs around empty tables, browning plants, and an unmanned help desk in the middle. It was eerie and unsettling to see a place that is usually so full of people completely empty.

With no one there to tell me I couldn't, I broke into a full run, silently reciting each step of the directions I'd been given at the check-in desk moments before on how to get to the Saperstein Critical Care Tower. *Take the double doors on the right, go outside, walk straight through the next set of double doors, curve around to the left, through another set of double doors you'll find an elevator bank. Take it to the sixth floor. Your husband is in room 602.*

I would do this walk almost every day for the next twelve weeks; each turn and step became something my body could do on autopilot. The walk took only five minutes, but this day, the first day, it felt like I would never get there. My body was tense, my stomach in knots, and my heart tight in my chest.

The sunlight glared in my eyes as I flung open the doors to go outside. It was April 18, another beautiful day in Los Angeles—the kind of day the three of us should be in Coldwater Canyon Park, with Nick pushing Elvis on a swing while I snapped photos. We should be headed to the beach, packing up a cooler with equal parts baby food and rosé and making family memories, or walking through Laurel Canyon with Elvis strapped to Nick's chest, or going to check on the progress of our new house on Love Street. We should be anywhere but here.

I finally arrived at the Saperstein tower—the words INTENSIVE CARE UNIT in bold, white letters across the front. I could read them perfectly, but at the same time they seemed like a foreign language. The last time we were in a hospital together was almost a year ago, for Elvis's birth. The maternity ward is full of new life, tears of joy, and smiles—I knew the ICU would be a very different experience.

Fluorescent lights replaced the sun as I entered. Cold replaced the warmth. I caught my breath as I encountered yet another abandoned desk. I fidgeted with my visitor's badge as I waited for the elevator—this little piece of plastic, which I had fought so hard to get, would finally allow me to visit my husband after eighteen days of being apart.

The hospital had called that morning. Every time the phone rang that month, everything stopped. We all froze, everything fell silent, and I held my breath as the medical staff delivered the news to me. I never knew what they were going to say. In the last two weeks, Nick had been admitted to the ICU, put on a ventilator, and placed in a medically in-duced coma. He had tested positive for COVID-19, gotten an infection, gone into septic shock, died for two minutes on the table, been resusci-tated, put on a machine called extracorporeal membrane oxygenation (ECMO for short) to save his life, and then gotten a blood clot in his right leg. Clots are a risk of ECMO; the machine that saves you can also destroy you.

Nick had internal bleeding, so they could not put him on blood thinners. But blood thinners were essential to breaking up the clot and getting blood flowing to the bottom half of his leg. His leg was turning black, slowly dying, and causing further trauma to his body. They had tried a small surgery—a fasciotomy procedure—to release the pressure caused by the clot, but it hadn't worked. For the last three days, the doctors had warned they might need to amputate Nick's right leg; it could potentially cause damage to the rest of his body if they didn't. Now I had to make a choice, but there was no real choice to make: it was his leg or his life. I chose his life.

"What time can you come in?" the nurse had asked me.

I almost dropped the phone when she said it. I asked every day, but the hospital had told me over and over again that I would not be allowed to come see him; they had said it again that very morning as I cried on the other end of the phone. The hospital was closed to visitors. This call, just an hour later, took my breath away—the head nurse suddenly asking, "When are you coming in?"

Right this very second!

They needed me to sign a consent form in order to do the surgery, and because of Nick's state there was a high risk he would not survive the amputation. It's hospital policy to allow family to visit prior to a surgery like this, just in case it's goodbye.

I had dropped everything and run out the door, leaving my half-eaten eggs and coffee behind on the table. My brother put Elvis, still in his pajamas, into the car, and we were driving five minutes later. The streets of Los Angeles were so empty under the Safer at Home emergency order that the drive, which ordinarily would take at least half an hour, took only ten minutes.

The shock of the sudden car trip when he should have been eating an early lunch caused Elvis to go into tears, so to keep him happy we put on his favorite song—"Can't Take My Eyes Off of You."

You're just too good to be true . . .

★   ★   ★

I sang this song to Elvis every day when he was in my womb. Nick would put a hand on my belly to feel his little kicks while I did. All Nick wanted was to be a dad. Elvis instantly calmed at the sound of it, and I looked back at my beautiful baby boy's reflection in the mirror. He was staring out the window—now calm and content—watching the world pass by his big, brown eyes. Nick's eyes. I felt so thankful that he would never remember any of this, and also so sad that if anything went wrong today, he would never remember his dad. Nick hadn't been able to kiss him, or me, goodbye when I dropped him off at the hospital eighteen days before. It was too much of a risk. So he shrugged, and waved, from six feet away. That had been our last goodbye.

The elevator opened, a right turn at the hallway, and there were the doors. I could see him through the glass immediately, lying in his corner room off to the left. I had been strong today until this point—I had accepted that this had to happen and believed it would be the thing that would finally start to change his progress for the better. But with that first glimpse of him, I crumbled. I saw for the first time what COVID-19 had done to Nick. Tears streamed down my face as I took it all in.

I was handed a box of tissues that I emptied in two minutes. My surgical mask was soaked through with tears instantly, and I had to replace it repeatedly over the next hour. As time went on, bodies moved around him, preparing him for surgery as quickly as possible. But for me, it was happening in slow motion. Standing next to the glass looking in, I couldn't believe it was real. I'd never felt so sick or helpless in my life. That was my husband in there, *my husband*. I couldn't hug him, or comfort him, or pray with him, or tell him how much I loved him.

His face was barely visible under the mess of tubes, lines, and machines around him. Three giant towers surrounded his bed, lit up and flickering like skyscrapers at night. He was still asleep, but his eyelids were too weak to fully close. I could see his eyes, eerily half open. He looked nothing like the man I had dropped off just eighteen days ago. Doctors and nurses in full PPE moved around him and slipped in and out of the room. Wearing a mask and gloves, I was allowed only as far as the glass wall outside his room, but each time someone opened the door to enter or exit, I screamed as loud I could:

"I LOVE YOU, NICK!"

"IT'S AMANDA, HONEY!"

"I'M HERE!"

I just wanted him to hear me.

I wanted him to know he wasn't alone.

I wanted him to wake up.

one

The Los Angeles stay-at-home order began March 19—the evening of my thirty-eighth birthday. We had been back from New York for just two days and weren't prepared for lockdown. We knew it was coming; other big cities around the world were shutting down, and city officials were projecting the number of cases in LA to be high, but we hadn't been able to go to the grocery store or prepare for anything.

So our friends had stocked our refrigerator in LA with anything they could find at the now-empty grocery stores. We had Lactaid because there wasn't regular milk, Stouffer's French Bread Pizza, instant potatoes, fried wonton chips, packages of frozen gnocchi, and a beef roast. It was a strange mix of things—most of which I would not usually eat—but we had enough to survive for a couple of days while we figured out life in quarantine. Our first night home, we put Elvis to bed, popped frozen pizzas in the oven, and opened a bottle of wine.

Nick felt terrible that there was nothing he could do for me for my birthday. My family always celebrates birthdays big, and he kept apologizing that I had to spend my birthday in quarantine, with nothing to do. For once, I didn't care. There was nothing to do and nowhere to go anyway. I kept telling him I was just glad we were together and safe. All I needed was my two men.

Several of our best friends live in Laurel Canyon, so we did a socially distanced birthday party with toasts and a surprise birthday cake from Magnolia Bakery that our friends had had the foresight to order a few days before. It was in the middle of that little party that we heard the news: Los Angeles was in lockdown for the next month.

We put Elvis to bed, and Nick made me his veggie gnocchi because it was the only option. He continuously apologized for serving veggie gnocchi on my birthday because it wasn't special—we ate it five nights a week! But to me, it always was. I cleaned my plate, but he picked at his. He wasn't that hungry, he said; he was feeling tired. I finished his plate—I couldn't let my birthday gnocchi go to waste. It was a strange birthday, but I didn't care. I didn't need a present, I told Nick; we had a brand-new home that we needed to spend every dime renovating.

"As soon as things are back to normal, I'm going to throw you the best birthday party," he kept saying.

I'd told him not to get me a gift, but he did give me a birthday card, and inside he wrote,

> I know this wasn't the day you wanted or deserve. Thank you for keeping your heart full and staying positive. Makes me love you even more. Elvis and I are so lucky. Thank you for being you.

That card, the last thing he gave me on our last normal day together, was the closest piece of paper I found when I first scrambled to write down the hospital's phone number. I grabbed the card and scribbled the number across the back. It stayed by the phone until the end, and I saw it each time I answered a call from the hospital.

We were still so exhausted from being in New York, so we crawled in bed early. That was the last time I slept beside my husband. I should have snuggled him harder.

Over the next two days, Nick continued to say he was really tired, exhausted, in fact, even after doing nothing. He repeatedly had to "go lie down for a minute." Each time he ended up taking a three- to four-hour nap. It did seem a little odd to me, but we had also just spent two weeks in New York, packing up our entire apartment. We had been through a lot physically, emotionally, and even mentally while trying to decide whether it was safe to fly back to LA. We were jet-lagged and exhausted. When Nick first said he was feeling fatigued on Friday morning, I thought, *Yeah—me, too.*

COVID was in the back of our minds at this point, of course. It was on everyone's mind.

But he had none of the symptoms.

He had no preexisting conditions.

He was forty-one years old.

We watched the news every evening, like everyone else in the world. It was the first time in modern history when everyone, everywhere, was going through the same thing. The whole world panicked, and changed, and then completely froze. We all went from living our busy, hectic, vastly different lives to all spending our days confined inside, with nothing to do and nowhere to go. We found ourselves glued to the news— just waiting for more information. What else was there to do? In the beginning, they were reporting that COVID was only affecting older people or people with respiratory issues. If you didn't have a fever or a cough, you didn't have COVID. That information seemed reputable. "Tired" wasn't a symptom. It was a daily reassurance that Nick was safe.

I was tired, too. We had a baby—I hadn't slept properly in eight months. I had just been in New York teaching dance-based fitness classes and running all over the city for work. I would have loved a day to lie on the couch and sleep. Nick could get into moods when he'd be a little depressed and would just lie around if he wasn't working, so I thought it was just that, exaggerated by the weirdness of the world at that moment. Everyone's life had just changed massively. For Nick, his show *Rock of Ages* had been canceled, all his work had come to a halt, and we couldn't go do anything fun. He was an extrovert—he loved to be out and around people. Everyone was processing the enormous change that was happening around the world, and a lot of people were battling depression as a result. His behavior seemed normal, all things considered.

I feel awful now, because at the time, I felt a little frustrated. He was just sleeping all day, and I was alone doing everything for Elvis, for the house, and for our family. I remember thinking, *Okay, I guess you're just going to sleep then*, and snapping a photo of him to send to my sisters poking fun at him. "This is Nick in quarantine."

I'm not one to idle. Despite being tired and confined, I had a business to run, and that business was currently the only thing bringing in money. I had just started a subscription series for my classes, so people could work out at home. But I had to create and film new content for it continuously in order to keep it generating income.

Nick was well enough to watch Elvis for an hour so that I could film a workout for it, or do a live workout with my friend Aimee Song. I was trying to think of ways to keep my business afloat and my body moving. I wanted Nick to do the same, but even after just watching Elvis for an hour, he was so tired he needed to sleep.

After a couple of days of this, I was convinced he needed to get some fresh air, get his body moving and mind going. So I gave him a training session one day, then made him go with me on a walk the next. He would sleep most of the day, but we had lunch and dinner together, and I noticed he was lethargic while moving between the bedroom and the kitchen. He definitely had a decrease in appetite, which was also strange for him. He was not one to turn down a cheese plate or a nice glass of wine. He still could taste and smell, another sign to me that he did not have COVID. The news was now reporting the loss of both as a new symptom.

For a few days, I saw what our life in quarantine might have been like. Together in the cabin with Elvis, taking walks through the Canyon, working out together in the driveway, eating dinner in every night. Before all this, our life had been pretty hectic most of the time. I trained in the morning, and Nick was at the show every night. I had initially thought—like many people—maybe this downtime would be nice for us. All that time together, all that time with Elvis while he's so young.

On the sixth day of his extreme fatigue, I asked him to change Elvis's diaper. He was in the bedroom, and I was in the kitchen when I heard a loud thump. I ran in to find Nick sprawled across the floor. When a six-foot-five-inch, 225-pound man falls to the ground, it makes quite a boom.

"What happened?" I asked, still stunned to have found him on the floor.

"I fainted, I guess," he replied.

"Have you ever fainted like that before?" I asked.

"No, I haven't."

"We're going to Urgent Care now. Get dressed," I said.

This was the first time I was a little scared. Something was definitely off with Nick, but still, there was no cough, no fever, no body aches. I hadn't heard of anyone young going into the hospital just because he was tired. Looking back, everyone who felt unwell in any way during that month was thinking the same thing . . . *Do I have this virus?*

Nick was convinced that he did.

I wasn't allowed inside the Urgent Care with him, and because LA was shut down, there was nothing for me to do but wait. I had no idea how long this would take, but after thirty minutes, with a baby in the car, you need to get creative. I put Elvis in the baby carrier and started doing a workout in the parking lot utilizing my Volvo SUV. The other two people in the parking lot looked at me like I was a crazy lady as I ran circles around my car and did wall squats using my car door. Elvis was giggling away. Used to the "mama and me" workouts I taught before quarantine, he thought it was a game.

A couple of hours later, Nick finally emerged from the Urgent Care. "Well, I don't have the flu—that test came back negative," he said. "They refused to test me for COVID because I don't have any of the symptoms, and I haven't been around anyone that was positive. So they took an X-ray of my lungs, and they think I have pneumonia."

Under normal circumstances, we would have been terrified, but we honestly felt a bit relieved. "Phew," we sighed. "Not COVID!" They sent us home with medication and an inhaler and told Nick to recover there. If he wasn't feeling better by Monday, he was to come back.

Back home, we started to keep our distance from each other, mainly because of Elvis. The medication was supposed to kick in and help him over the weekend, but Nick just grew more and more fatigued, and his breathing had gotten bad. He also developed a cough—but it wasn't a dry one. It was terrible sounding, very phlegmy. The guest bedroom area looked like a mini–hospital room. It was covered in tissues, medications, Pedialyte, Ensure bottles, cups, and clothes.

I was keeping our families and friends updated, and no one was really alarmed. At this point, we still all thought, *Even if Nick does have COVID, he'll be okay.* By Sunday night, though, we were worried. He was supposed to be getting better, but he was only getting worse. We called a doctor we knew through a friend and described all his symptoms. "If his breathing gets worse, go to the hospital right away," he said.

I went to bed that night, scared, praying for Nick to wake up feeling better.

The next morning, we decided to go to the emergency room. Nick was hesitant; he knew he would have to be there alone, and going to the hospital is never fun. Now we were in the middle of the COVID crisis, and it felt extra dangerous. I told him to get dressed, and I would make him breakfast.

It took him thirty minutes to take the few steps from the bedroom to the kitchen table, and he took just two bites of oatmeal.

I dropped him off in front of Cedars-Sinai an hour later. We weren't sure where to go or which part of the hospital was open, so I left him on the corner and he started walking toward the hospital.

"I'll just stay nearby with Elvis. Call me when you want me to pick you up," I said.

We didn't hug or kiss goodbye.

We couldn't.

He didn't say goodbye to Elvis, which breaks my heart every time I think about it.

It was clear he had something, but we weren't thinking that there was any possibility of his being admitted. We thought that I was dropping him off for an hour, maybe two.

I had no idea that would be the last time I would ever see him as *him*.

He was never the same again. He woke up, but he never really came back.

In a crowded room of people, you couldn't miss Nick. He was six feet five inches, with dark hair and dark eyes . . . and an undeniable presence.

The first time I saw him was on day one of the reading for the new Woody Allen and Susan Stroman musical, *Bullets over Broadway*. This is the earliest stage of a Broadway show: the reading. A cast of actors sits in a rehearsal room with the entire team and reads through the script. It's the first moment you hear the lines read aloud and can start to imagine the show coming to life. Everyone in the theater world was talking about this show already; it was going to be the next huge hit. Just being in that little room at 890 Broadway, you felt special. For an actor, a show like this is a dream job because it means stability. If you are in a hit show, you can breathe; you know you have a paycheck for at least the next year.

Broadway is a small world. Everyone knows everyone or knows of everyone, but I had never heard of Nick. I don't remember our first conversation; I just remember looking up at him while we were talking and thinking, *Wow, he is so tall.* At five feet ten, that's not a thought I've had very often.

I was ecstatic that I had been asked to do this reading. Being asked to do a reading for a Broadway show is like being asked to join a secret club or being given a pass to the VIP section. A reading happens before auditions for a show officially begin, so as an actor, it feels like a small "in." It is also a chance to show the director what you've got, and if you do well, there's a good chance you'll get to be a part of the Broadway company. So as an actor vying for the role, you come to the reading with guns blazing. I was dressed to the nines each day, along with everyone else. I was alert at all times; even when I was not reading or needed at that moment, I was sitting up, back straight and eyes open, with a big smile, just in case.

Nick was reading for the iconic role of Cheech, the key supporting role under the main character, David, who was played by Zach Braff. I was in the female ensemble and felt right at home. I had worked with Susan Stroman many times before, so I knew the drill. There is an unspoken decorum and order with her: show up ready to go, ladies with a bright red lip, men looking sharp. Lead roles sit in the front, ensemble behind them. Everyone should have their script and music in hand and stay on the edge of their seats. Her motto is: "Full out with great conviction!" She's inspiring to work for and makes you want to work hard.

Clearly, Nick hadn't gotten the memo.

He arrived each day in dirty gym clothes, sat in the back, far away from everyone, reclining in his seat and looking as if he couldn't care less. He was a loner, talking to people only during our allotted ten-minute equity breaks and not making any effort to be involved.

"Does this guy realize he's auditioning for a lead role in the biggest show on Broadway?" I wondered. His behavior perplexed me.

At the end of the week in a reading, you do a mock performance of the script for potential producers and the entire team. It was a huge success. Afterward, I stood in the lobby talking to Nick. To my surprise, he had been great in the reading! I was wondering if he was going to book this job when the set designer came out and interrupted our conversation.

"So do you have your driver's license?" he asked.

Cheech drove a car onstage in the show. Nick had just booked the job.

Later, when we were dating, he explained his behavior to me.

"Amanda," he reasoned, "Cheech is a gangster, a hit man! He would never sit in the front row, waiting on the edge of his seat, giddy and grateful to be there. He wants nothing to do with this show or anyone in it."

He was auditioning from the moment he walked in. He arrived each day playing the part of Cheech. I laughed through the "aha" moment. "Well, honey, that's what makes you such a great actor."

He knew what he was doing all along; he always did.

The next time I saw him, I was naked, aside from a pelt of fur. I had been asked to model the costumes for the show, so I was with the wardrobe team in our rehearsal space. They were pinning fur onto my body when the elevator door opened, and there was Nick.

"Oh," I said, and he blushed!

"I'm here for my tap lesson," he said.

"I'm demoing the costumes for the show," I said.

We awkwardly waved and went back to our business, but Nick told me later that he would never forget the image of me standing there, naked, and wrapped in fur.

I knew all the girls in the show already and had worked with most of them before. The dressing room quickly becomes like a grown-up slumber party. When we started rehearsals for *Bullets over Broadway*, I remember hearing continuously, "That Nick guy is pretty cute!"

"Really?" I'd respond. "I mean, I guess so."

I wasn't looking. I was happily married. Or I thought I was.

At the time, I was married to an actor I had met several years earlier in another show, my first one on Broadway, the Beach Boys musical *Good Vibrations*. We fell in love young—I was only twenty-three when we met—got married two years later, and had been living together in New York for the past six years. It is both difficult and fantastic to be in a relationship with another actor because you experience the same ups and downs. It's wonderful when they can help prepare you for your audition, reassure you when you're cut, and understand your exact feelings of success and failure. But it's an added challenge when you both end up out of work, or on tour. Right when I got the part in *Bullets over Broadway*, he got the role of Elder Price in the touring company of *Book of Mormon*. It meant a year apart for us, at least, but as an actor, you can't turn those roles down. It also meant insurance and two stable paychecks. As a young married couple, you can't turn those things down either.

By this point, my husband was two months into his national tour. Tour life is hard because it isn't grounded in reality. You are a professional, an adult, yet you have no responsibilities, no expenses, and no schedule all day until your show in the evening. You are in a different city every couple of weeks, so there's no home to maintain or family to visit, or mundane activities to attend to. You spend your days alone or with the other cast members, and then do the show. After the show, you typically hit up the local bar, have way too many drinks, and stumble back to your hotel room.

This routine is the perfect recipe for disaster. I had done three national tours in my professional career, so I knew firsthand what my husband was getting into when he started in December 2014, and I was a little worried. He was a social butterfly, loved everyone and was loved by everyone. He was always the life of the party. We had been thinking of starting a family soon, and going on tour was the total opposite of that. *Bullets over Broadway* was set to begin in January. We would both be insanely busy for the next several months and on opposite sides of the country. I knew in my gut that something was going to go wrong, and I think he did, too. Before he left for tour, my now ex-husband shook Nick's hand and said, "Take care of Amanda for me while I'm away."

The next several months didn't go well. The long distance between us took a tremendous toll on our marriage and magnified any existing problems we had. We worked at our marriage and tried to reconcile, but, unfortunately, it became clear that what he needed and what I needed were completely different. We decided to separate and then eventually divorce. I had been married for seven years, and this was not easy.

Even though I knew it was the right thing, I never imagined myself getting divorced. I never wanted that for my life; no one does, and it's a hard reality to face. I felt embarrassed and ashamed. I felt like I had failed at the thing most important to succeed at. I felt as if I had just lost everything: my best friend, husband, and the family I had envisioned us having. I was a mess.

Bullets over Broadway opened at the same time, so I was able to distract myself with the show and the new friends I made in the cast. Your cast becomes like a little family while you're in a show. With my husband now gone, I needed an adoptive family. I remember one night after the show going to a bar next to the theater with the cast. Nick was sitting at the bar alone, so I took the stool next to him, and we had our first real conversation.

It was one of those conversations that sparks a connection, a real bond. We ended up talking for hours—it felt like a movie scene where the time passes in slow motion for two characters, while the world all around them continues moving at its usual pace. I hadn't talked to anyone much at that point, but I confessed a lot to Nick that night. I told him about my marriage, what was happening, and how I felt. He felt safe and comforting and just listened; he was a great listener. He opened up about his previous relationship, which had some odd similarities. People came in and out of the scene around us, but we kept coming back to this deep conversation until we suddenly realized it was two o'clock in the morning.

Later I walked to the subway, thinking, *Oh no. Do I like this guy?*

I kept myself busy all day, every day, so that I wouldn't dwell on the sadness. I taught fitness classes from eight in the morning until noon, surrounded by energy and music. I was so invested in helping people become more fit that I was able to get my mind off my problems. I walked out of the studio, smiling and happy, full of endorphins. Then I had to go to my Broadway show each night. As we say in theater, "The show must go on!"

Singing and dancing saved my life. I got to disguise my sorrow with stage makeup, wigs, and beautiful costumes and hear people cheering in the audience.

After the show, we would all go out, and I'd drink my sorrows away.

It was the same every day, and it was how I got by. And in the middle of all that, Nick and I started dating.

For a while I didn't tell anyone I was going through a divorce—as I said, Broadway is a small world. So since no one really knew, Nick and I had to date secretly for a time. I didn't want word to get out, and he didn't want to look as if he was seeing a married woman.

If it weren't for Nick, I don't think I would have gotten through my divorce. It's strange who you end up feeling you can talk to when things go wrong. My friends were there for me, but I couldn't talk to them. I spoke to my family every day; my mom was a rock star. But I needed someone I could say things to who didn't know all about my marriage and didn't feel as if he knew all about me. I was so grateful to him every day during that time. I still am. He never judged me or questioned me. He just listened and held me while I cried day after day about what was happening. He became my boyfriend and best friend simultaneously.

He lived in Washington Heights at the time, all the way north— 190th Street on the A train. I was in East Harlem until I moved to my own studio on West Sixty-Eighth Street. Our early years were fun and carefree, like a college relationship.

Bullets over Broadway was not the success it was supposed to be. It closed that August, after only 156 performances. We all mourned the loss of the show we loved doing, the jobs we thought were secure, and the little family we had formed. So we stayed close, a small group of us. Nick and I continued to spend time with Preston Boyd, who is now Elvis's godfather, and Zach Braff, who became one of our best friends.

With the show canceled, Nick and I had a lot of time to spend together "up north," as I called it. We were both technically unemployed, so a lot of nights we bought a cheap bottle of wine, and Nick made us a meal of sliced tomatoes and mozzarella. We would sit on the floor of his studio, picnic-style, and talk for hours about anything and everything. Those are some of my favorite memories. In every place we lived in afterward, we made sure to have "tomato and mozz" nights.

Everyone told me that it was too soon to be dating someone. That I needed time alone to heal and figure things out—Nick said that more than anyone. But I always told them that being with Nick made me happy, and at that time, I needed to do things that made me happy.

My parents came to New York that fall and I wanted them to meet

Nick, but I was very nervous about it. They had been so close with my ex-husband, it felt weird to be introducing someone new to them. How could anyone else ever fit in?

My sisters Ali and Anna lived in New York at the time and had already met Nick a few times, so I decided we should all go out to dinner the first night my parents were in town. My sisters would be good buffers and would help make Nick feel more comfortable. Nick knew at this point that our families were very different: his family has few filters and will openly talk about everything. I essentially grew up in a modern-day Brady Bunch, and my mom still spells out anything she considers a bad word, including "penis." Nick was a little worried about what was okay to say and not say, do and not do. We got a big round table at a cozy restaurant, and as soon as we sat down, my sisters began their prank to cut the tension.

"So," Alison began, "whenever we're all together for a meal, we play a game called 'Go Around the Table.' You have to go around the table and say what you love about the person to your left. I'll start!"

And we went around the table . . .

Ali was next to my mom, my mom was next to my dad, my dad was next to me, I was next to Nick, and Nick was next to Anna.

He was up . . .

"Anna," he said, "I really like what you did with your hair tonight— it's very Maid Marian!"

She had it parted in the middle, half up, half down, with two little braids connecting in the back.

We all burst out laughing. "We weren't going to make you actually do it!" we said.

But his answer, and enthusiasm, had been perfect.

I think I knew right then he would fit in just fine.

Still, Nick and I were very different people. Nick always said "too different." We didn't see the world, marriage, and family the same. Nick would stay out till five a.m., never wanting to leave a party, and I wanted to be tucked into bed by ten o'clock. Nick had had a wild past, and I was as straitlaced as someone could be. Nick loved music and would spend hours discovering artists. I only made playlists for my cardio classes, curated from the Top 40. Nick would spend hours lying in bed, looking at the ceiling, and I had to go, go, go—all day long.

We didn't see religion the same either. I had been raised Christian, and my faith was at the root of every choice I made. I wanted my kids to go to Sunday school and a husband who would pray with me at night. Nick was not a believer. He wasn't an atheist; he felt as if God is in us all, that we are God. He had never read the Bible and didn't particularly enjoy church unless there was a fantastic choir. He definitely didn't want to raise a child in any specific faith. We had many arguments about it.

We had our ups and downs. We fought. We broke up twice.

How could this ever work? I thought.

We love each other, but it just isn't meant to be.

We broke up the last time the following summer, and it seemed like for good. The separation felt right until Nick's dad got sick with cancer. I found myself thinking of him all the time, sending him photos of places in New York City that reminded me of us while he was home in Hamilton. We were broken up yet still very much together. When he came back from Canada, he asked me to train him. He wanted to get into shape, take better care of himself, be in better shape for auditions. Actors are always worried about their appearance.

"I'll pay you," he said. He was not asking for any favors.

"Oh gosh," I replied. "Absolutely not! Let's start tomorrow."

It was the *Bullets over Broadway* reading all over again, except this time he was vying for a different role. He showed up in new workout clothes from Old Navy that he had purchased for the occasion—I knew this outfit was not from his closet. He was ready to impress.

I gave him my instructions, started the music, and cautiously handed him the jump rope.

We had tried before to get him to jump rope, and he could never do it. It always frustrated him, and no matter what I did or said he could not get the hang of it. I was prepared for yet another disaster.

He started with a slow basic jump that was good.

Then he got a little faster and was perfect!

I couldn't believe it. What had I said or done this time that worked? Suddenly, he started doing tricks—cross-jumps, and double-unders!

What is happening? I thought.

"Nick, this is amazing! How are you suddenly so good?" I asked

He then confessed: before visiting his dad in the hospital each morning, he would wake up early and go to the gym to teach himself how to jump rope so he could win me back.

He knew what he was doing. He nailed the audition, yet again. My heart melted, and from that day on, we never looked back.

A couple of months later, we found a fantastic one-bedroom apartment one block from my studio on West Sixty-Ninth Street, right across from Magnolia Bakery, and decided to move in together.

The night we signed the lease, we sat in Lincoln Center looking at the Met, celebrating with ice cream from a Mister Softee ice-cream truck. Nick kept saying, "I can't wait to explore our new neighborhood," which made me laugh because it was only one block from my current studio, where we already spent most of our time. We celebrated our first night in the apartment with a picnic on the floor: "tomato and mozz" and a cheap bottle of wine.

It was the nicest apartment Nick or I had ever rented, and we were so happy there. Going from our two studios on opposite sides of Manhattan to a one-bedroom together was life-changing. We had eight hundred square feet for the first time—and three whole closets. We felt like kings. It got great light and looked over Sixty-Ninth Street. There was room for a kitchen table, a couch, and a coffee table in the living room. Nick made a little corner into his music nook with his keyboard, guitars, record player, and vinyl. Our kitchen was long and narrow, with tons of cabinet space. It was enormous by New York standards, which meant we could both be in there cooking at the same time.

It was our first home. We grew together in this apartment. We became successful in this apartment, got engaged and married in this apartment, and found out we were pregnant in this apartment. Later my sister Alison moved into an apartment a floor above us. It felt like our own little slice of the Upper West Side.

I had been a New Yorker for fifteen years at that point. I moved there in 2000 to attend the American Musical and Dramatic Academy, and I wanted to perform on Broadway and become a Radio City Rockette. My career took off when I graduated and booked a national tour of *42nd Street*.

I toured for ten months all over America, and I was living my dream. I had seen *42nd Street* ten times on Broadway, sitting in the "student seats" during college, and I couldn't believe that my first professional job was in this show. Each week was a new city, and I'd explore and write my parents a postcard describing all the things I was doing. They kept them all, and I have them to this day. I was twenty years old; it was the perfect time to be on the road, carefree. Doing that show cemented my love for performing.

But this lifestyle is exhausting, and as you get older, the instability of it becomes scarier. You have no control over whether the show you book will be a sensation or a total flop. One week you're living your dream, dancing on a Broadway stage, and the next you're unemployed, willing to dress up as Cinderella for a child's birthday party in order to make an extra $300. So fifteen years later, when *Bullets over Broadway* closed, I was devastated. I was going through my divorce at the same time, and I felt I had no control over anything in my life. Nothing was mine; nothing was certain. I wanted a family. I wanted a home. How would I ever achieve those things if I stayed on this path of off-and-on employment?

I had spent the past fifteen years performing at Radio City, on Broadway, and in theaters around the world. I had been in a few films, and on television. I had danced in the Macy's Thanksgiving Day Parade. I had worked with every director I dreamed of working with. It felt like I was ready to move on.

Teaching fitness classes was my side hustle at the time, but I had started to become passionate about it. I loved helping people; I loved the endorphin boost. I loved creating new ways to challenge myself. The studio I taught at was mostly dance cardio, but one day I was training a private client and handed her a jump rope to start warming up. I started jumping with her, and I had a thought: *What if we don't put this rope down. What could I create with it to make a full-body class?* By the time the session ended, and we were both exhausted, I knew I was on to something.

For a while, I kept one toe in the performing world as a safety net. I could go back if this didn't work out. But after a year, my business was growing fast, and it didn't make sense for me to focus on anything else. Nick encouraged me to keep going. He was so supportive of my business and of my leaving the theater to become a CEO of my own brand. I was incredibly grateful that he took that leap of faith in me; it made believing in the end goal easier.

I started teaching several times a week at New York's newest workout hot spot, Studio B, and I was booked solid for privates, sometimes five in a day. I was so happy to be running my own business, to be in control. When I was teaching a sold-out class, it felt a lot like I was performing. I was at the front, smiling and dancing, and in a way it was like my own stage. It made giving up theater a lot easier; I felt I had a piece of it still.

Nick had moved to New York from Toronto to pursue acting and be on Broadway. He had spent years performing in various bands in Canada, working on music with his friends, and he always wanted to be a rock star. He had spent several years performing on cruise ships and arrived in New York fresh off the boat, with a few thousand dollars to his name. Acting had been mostly a struggle for him. Being so tall and such a specific type, he was "right" for only a few roles on Broadway. His first big break in New York was booking *The Toxic Avenger*, a hit off-Broadway show with a cult following. He played a seven-foot mutant freak with superhuman powers—that's showbiz, kid!

Bullets over Broadway was huge for Nick. He was taking real estate classes when he booked the reading, something a lot of actors do when they feel like they might leave the business. At some point, you start to think, *I need a steady income if this isn't going to work.*

After years of struggling, he was nominated for a Tony Award for Cheech. After a Tony nomination, everything changes. He got the role of Earl in *Waitress* opposite Jesse Mueller and then left that show to take the lead role of Sonny in *A Bronx Tale*. He opened the show and was met outside the stage door each night by fans wanting him to sign their Playbill.

Eight years after he arrived in New York, he had done it. He was a star.

So much had changed for us in a year. We were both more successful than we ever had been before, we had a home together, and our relationship was rock solid. I would spend the whole day teaching for my business, and he would do his show. A lot of nights, I would meet him after *A Bronx Tale* was over, and we would go for fun, expensive late-night dinner dates around Manhattan. Our favorite was Friday nights at Del Frisco's. We'd cuddle in a big leather banquet, drink a great bottle of wine, and eat a huge steak dinner at eleven o'clock at night. That is what's special about living in New York City.

"So, when do you think you might want to get married?" I asked Nick one night. I'll never forget his response:

"I'm in no rush. I think we should take some time, travel the world together, and, you know—if that goes well—maybe get engaged after?"

"Nick," I replied, "when is that supposed to happen? I'm thirty-five—I want a baby, and a family, and a home! I didn't move in with you to hang out for a while, travel the world, and *maybe, 'if that goes well,'* get married!"

He proposed two months later, the morning after my birthday, on a little trip to Woodstock, New York. Six months later, we got married; a year after that we found out we were pregnant; and four months after Elvis was born, we bought our first house. It was a lot of massive life changes in a short period of time, but it was everything I had dreamed of.

two

On March 30, I pulled away from Cedars-Sinai and parked the car on Third Street. It seemed silly to drive all the way home; I didn't think Nick would be there for more than an hour. I used to walk up and down that street all the time when I first lived in LA while performing on the *42nd Street* national tour. I smiled as I passed a restaurant Nick took me to on a date night shortly after we'd first arrived in LA the previous September. I kept walking until I got to The Grove, a big outdoor shopping area. The Grove is like Disneyland; it has perfectly manicured lawns, twinkle lights, beautiful fountains, and a retro feel.

Los Angeles was empty, so I was the only person there. It was the strangest feeling, as if there had been an apocalypse. It was a beautiful day, and the music was still playing through the speakers. I sat on the lawn with Elvis, waiting, and it was beautiful. The fountains were on, and happy music was playing:

Volare, oh, oh
Cantare, oh, oh, oh, oh

It was a sign! Whenever Nick made me his gnocchi, we would put on an Italian playlist from Spotify, and that song was the first one up. It's also always playing in Capri, where we spent part of our honeymoon. I sat on the perfectly manicured green lawn, playing with Elvis and singing our song, thinking, *Everything will be okay! Volare! It's a sign!*

But the rest of the day unfolded just as oddly as that morning had: hourly updates from Nick that grew increasingly strange and scary.

First, he called to tell me they were going to keep him for a few hours. "They think I might have it, so they did a COVID test, but we won't have those results for a few days. You might want to go home, darling," he said.

A couple hours later, he called again, telling me that they had decided to keep him overnight.

I wished I could go back to the hospital right then, but I couldn't. The restrictions were already in place, and Cedars was not allowing any visitors. When the phone rang at two a.m., I searched desperately for my phone in my half-awake state.

"Honey," Nick said, "they're taking me to the ICU. My organs aren't getting enough oxygen."

I was terrified, confused, and starting to panic. ICU? I have never had anyone I love in the ICU before; those three letters together sounded horrible.

He spent the whole next day in his hospital bed, on oxygen. We FaceTimed, but because of his breathing issues, he couldn't talk very long. They had done another COVID test, but the results weren't back yet. At home, I tried to do my regular routine with Elvis, but I was distracted. I felt so helpless. My husband was in the ICU, and I couldn't visit. I couldn't even talk to him.

I went to bed that night with my phone in my hand and Elvis cuddled next to me.

My phone rang at four in the morning.

"Honey," Nick said, "they want to put me on a ventilator."

I was in a daze, caught off guard, and I couldn't find the words even to respond.

"They have to put me in a medically induced coma so my body can rest. It should only be a few days, but I won't be able to talk to you anymore after this call. I'm scared," he said.

"I'm scared, too, honey," I whispered, trying not to wake up Elvis, "but it will be okay. I'm sure what the doctors are saying is the right thing. I'll take care of Elvis—don't worry about us. I love you," I said.

"I love you, too."

I didn't understand the seriousness of that decision. Neither did Nick.

April 1 at four a.m. was the last time I heard my husband's voice.

I could barely sleep for the rest of that night.

My friends generously offered to cover the cost of a private healthcare team to supplement the standard care provided by our medical plan. I didn't really understand what that meant, but because of that, he would now have an additional head doctor—Dr. Ng—on his case, working with the team in the ICU, so I started referring to Dr. Ng as "this rockstar doctor" when talking to my friends and family. This private healthcare team was also going to call me throughout his hospitalization and give me updates. They called me for the first time that afternoon and introduced me to Dr. Ng. He was indeed a rock star. He is one of the head pulmonary doctors at Cedars-Sinai and has a successful private practice as well. At the time, I didn't understand the full extent of my friends' gift; looking back now, though, I see that without it, everything would have been different. This was the first of many incredibly gracious acts, and I will be forever grateful to my friends who got Nick this level of care from day one.

It was Dr. Ng who first said on that call, "Despite two negative tests, I'm certain that this is COVID. His body is acting like he has this virus.

We'll do a third COVID test now that he's under because we'll be able to get deep into the lung cavities to get a true sample. We'll start treating him like he's COVID positive, so we'd like to start hydroxychloroquine. There's no way this isn't COVID."

At the time, it was all over the news that hydroxychloroquine was saving people's lives, so I felt relieved. I liked that Dr. Ng had the foresight to start treating Nick as if he was positive because it gave us the opportunity to get the drugs in him as soon as possible.

I was shocked and scared and decided to go on Instagram to share with my friends and social media community. What had happened to Nick in the past two weeks was something I felt people needed to know. What if other people sitting at home were just "tired"? What if other people believed what we had believed: "I'm young, I'll be fine—even if I get it." There were obviously other symptoms that weren't on the news.

Everyone had been saying young people weren't being affected.

I felt I needed to let people know this was real and dangerous. The story got shared on *Daily Mail* within an hour, and then appeared on People.com. Then it was suddenly everywhere. The support flooded in overnight. My best girlfriends in New York City immediately got on a Zoom with me, asking how they could help. They began sending me food every day. Nick's cast from *Rock of Ages* also came to my rescue, with daily Elvis walks so that I could work, sleep, shower, or cry. The producer would text me, asking me what he could bring me from the grocery store. My neighbors and close friends in the Canyon did socially distanced check-ins to see if I needed help. The support was incredible.

I began doing research. I needed to know what we were dealing with. When I have a problem, I'm the kind of person who likes to find the solution as soon as possible. So I made calls. I knew of some people in the Broadway community who had been hospitalized, spent four or five days in the ICU, and were now home. That brought me peace. It could be a scary few days, but he would be home. He was forty-one and healthy. I prayed and had faith that everything was going to be okay.

Elvis and I got into a rhythm at home alone. I would wake up and feed him breakfast, and we would play with his toys for a while. I FaceTimed with my mom and dad for a while after that so I wouldn't feel alone. Then a friend would come to take Elvis on a walk so that I could go live on Instagram to do a workout. With pending hospital bills and my husband unconscious, it felt more important than ever to keep my business afloat. We later began calling this team of people his Stroller Buddies.

Each day, I made videos of Elvis and me that I sent to Nick's phone.

Hi, Dada, it's day __, we miss you so much. Look what I am doing, Dada! Get home soon. We love you!"

I wanted Nick to wake up and feel like he was a part of each day he'd missed while sleeping.

In order to clean, shower, or get anything done, I would put Elvis in his crib and turn on *Elmo*. If that didn't last, I started doing full-on performances for him, dancing around the bedroom in my socks performing bits from Broadway shows I had been in. I would love to say that he looked impressed, but he was a hard sell. I was finding ways to entertain us both, to keep us smiling, cheerful, and positive.

In the afternoon, we'd crawl back into bed and take a nap from two to four. He would wake up and play, have dinner at six thirty, and then I'd put him to bed.

Once Elvis was down, I would call Nick's mom, Lesley, while cooking my dinner. She was in Toronto with Nick's whole family, so it was important that I kept them in the loop. The health-care team called me twice a day, so at night I always gave Lesley the daily report.

She and I remained very confident that Nick was going to be just fine and that he seemed to improve every day. Each day we got closer to their taking him off the ventilator, which meant he would wake up and come home! There was no reason to panic.

When I got off the phone with her, I would sit down with my dinner and FaceTime my little sister, Anna. She had just flown back from Europe and was alone in Ohio, isolated in a friend's empty house until it was safe to join my parents in theirs. We were both lonely and sad, so we would talk for an hour, sometimes more. She was one week into the Whole30 diet, and I was being sent amazing desserts and comfort food every night. We can always make each other laugh. She complained about how gross her homemade, sugar-free banana "nice cream" was while watching me slowly devour the gooey cookies that had shown up on my doorstep that day. These chats always helped the night end with a smile.

"I wish I could get out to you, Mandy," she said. "I wish I was allowed! I don't like that you're out there alone."

Neither did I.

I had not wanted to move to Los Angeles.

It was something we fought about, every day, for over a year before it finally happened. In 2018, Nick and I spent two months in LA, so that he could be there for pilot season and audition for roles on television. I taught classes so that I could become better known on the West Coast. After twenty years of living in New York, it was nice to escape the cold winter and spend a few months away from home.

We had such a great time, we came back to do the same thing in 2019. This little taste of La-La Land sold Nick completely. Elvis was due that June. He wanted a real home for our family, a yard for our dogs, and the chance to chase the music and acting opportunities he was confident were waiting for him in California.

He would always say, "I smell opportunity in Los Angeles. I've done everything I want to do in New York." He had been offered a role in *Rock of Ages*, opening on Hollywood Boulevard that fall, and he wanted to be somewhere he could work on his music. Los Angeles is where the music industry is based, and Laurel Canyon is the heart of it. The cherry on top was that Zach Braff had offered us his guesthouse in the Canyon, rent free, for as long as we needed it. The guesthouse even had a name—Brown Bear. That was reason enough for Nick to want to pack up our new family and move across the country.

We were different—remember? I felt the complete opposite. I loved spending a few weeks a year in LA, but I did not want to move permanently. I was pregnant. My parents had just retired and moved to New York City to be near Nick and Elvis and me, as well as my two sisters, who also lived in New York. In fact, I had found my parents an apartment across the hall from my own. My dad would knock on our door in the morning to let us know there were hot pancakes ready in his kitchen. My sister Ali was also about to have a baby, so I had a best friend to go through the stages of pregnancy and postpartum with. It was the first child for both of us, and every client, friend, and family member of mine confirmed, "You'll need help when you have your first baby." To leave New York with that kind of support system in place, my mom and dad just across the hall, seemed crazy.

I could imagine our life in New York with a baby; it was what I knew and had grown accustomed to. Los Angeles had traffic, and we would need a car. It was isolating and spread out. In Manhattan, you pop the baby in the stroller, and you head out for the day—no car, no traffic, no fuss. I had spent the last five years building my business from the ground up. I had steady clients and work and opportunities. I had friends with whom I had spent the previous twenty years and loved like family. We had a lease we couldn't break on a fully renovated two-bedroom on the Upper West Side one block from Central Park. Why in the world would we want to move right now?

We saw two different worlds and futures, but Nick would not shut up about California. Such a huge part of marriage is compromise and understanding. I knew that unless I agreed to go to LA and try it, he would never be happy. He had grown so negative about Manhattan that it affected his daily mood, and it was important to me that my husband be happy. We compromised, agreeing to have Elvis in New York in June, and then move to California in September. It gave me a few months with my family before we would have to say goodbye.

We had to sublet our apartment for the final six months of the lease, which felt like a nice security blanket to me. We could live in LA, but our home in New York would still be there with everything inside. It would sit waiting for us just in case things didn't work out.

On September 16, 2019, we left Manhattan with a newborn, two dogs, three guitars, and seven suitcases that contained as much of our life as we could pack up. We arrived in Los Angeles like *The Beverly Hillbillies*.

I cried the whole plane ride there. Nick was beaming brighter than the LA sunshine.

The next month was a daily battle for me. I was postpartum and emotional, and I cried every single day. Elvis was only three months old, so I was still getting the hang of the drastic change to our routine. So was Nick. He was an amazing dad, but a new one. He didn't know what to do when Elvis cried or fussed and would panic after just a few minutes.

"I think he wants you," he would say hesitantly, approaching me with his arms outstretched, a squirming Elvis, and a sheepish grin.

I was able to start teaching right away at the new Los Angeles location of Studio B, inside the Bandier store on Melrose. But it was new, and so was I, and it felt like no one knew or cared that we were there. My class numbers were dismal, so we lived off the income from a small number of private sessions. I felt like a failure. I had worked so hard to build a little empire in New York, and now I was starting from scratch all over again. But my priorities had shifted; Elvis was number one now. I could no longer spend eight hours a day training and making videos and attending events hoping to make connections to get my name out there. I had a son, and he came first.

Nick's show opening had been delayed because the theater wasn't ready. So he spent his days "working on his music." I now feel so guilty to say it, but I'll admit it: I didn't understand "his music." He had books of half-written songs and a slew of old bands he had created. He started spending all day recording and rewriting lyrics, and that studio time is expensive. We didn't have the money, and I didn't understand his end goal.

"He's too old to just suddenly become a rock star," I complained to Anna.

We had a fight about it when Nick explained his vision. If things took off, we would go on tour, play little gigs, and gain momentum. I looked at him, baffled, demanding to know how I, my business, a newborn baby, and two untrained Morkies were supposed to pack up, hit the road, and go on tour with him? I didn't want to be unsupportive, but it was not realistic. He was forty-one and a dad. He wasn't going to become a rock star overnight. We had to be practical.

The fighting made me feel even more lost and lonely, and I called my family every day while I was driving home from work, saying, "I just want to come back to New York."

Meanwhile, Nick was house shopping.

We knew that if we were going to stay in Los Angeles we wanted to live in Laurel Canyon. We loved the old-fashioned feel of the neighborhood and its historical significance in the music world. As we drove the streets, Nick would point out the former home of every notable person, every single time.

"That's Joni's house," he'd say as we passed.

"I know, babe," I'd reply.

Laurel Canyon was where all our closest friends lived. It also has one of the best schools in the city: Wonderland. A ten-out-of-ten rated elementary school where creativity is fostered. We wanted that education for Elvis and that community for our family. But because of all these perks, prices were high and out of our range. We had been watching the market for the last year. We had seen places smaller than our New York apartment come on the market at a price we could *maybe* afford, only to sell in an instant for several thousand dollars above asking. Our only chance was to find a bit of a fixer-upper and get to it before someone else did. Laurel Canyon is a tight-knit community, and we were in luck that we were already kind of a part of it. It allowed us to see FOR SALE signs first, and sometimes get the inside scoop from a neighbor.

We went to listing after listing, and most of them were terrible. Our budget didn't allow for the kind of home we wanted or the space we needed.

It was late October, and we had planned a fun family day with Elvis—a Halloween party in Culver City. As I was getting ready, Nick rushed in with a listing in his hand for an open house he just found and wanted us to visit: a three-bedroom, two-bathroom home behind our favorite restaurant, Pace. It was the perfect size and location. There were just a few photos, but you could see the living room got fantastic sunlight. It was listed at our maximum budget. It was a week before Halloween— this would be either a trick or a treat.

"Let's check it out," I agreed.

Elvis was Elvis for his first Halloween, obviously. I had found a cheap, polyester costume on Amazon of the famous white, studded suit and cape that even came with a beanie hat that looked like a head of dark, wavy hair. We walked into the house, and the first thing we saw, hanging above a piano, was a black-and-white photo of Elvis Presley in *Jailhouse Rock*.

I have always believed in signs. I pray to God every night for direction, and guidance, and patience, and understanding. I had been miserable in Los Angeles, desperate to go back to New York and be with my family, and hanging on to a sliver of hope that things wouldn't work out here and Nick would agree to go back to the East Coast. Buying a house would make Los Angeles home. It would change everything for good.

We kept looking around, individually, and came together upstairs. An entire shrine of Elvis memorabilia was displayed in a corner. It took the wind out of me. *Okay, Lord,* I thought, *I hear you.*

The house needed work. It was so small. One "bedroom" was actually a closet; the only one in the house. The bathroom and kitchen and entire downstairs would need to be gutted, and we couldn't afford that. So we would have to live in the upstairs to begin with, and convert the closet into a nursery for Elvis. The outside patio was a mess of cracked bricks and overgrown plants and trees that desperately needed a manicure.

I looked at Nick and said, "I hate to say this because I haven't been happy here, and I don't want to buy a house yet, and I don't think I want to live in Los Angeles. But this is our home."

Nick's smile was one of the best sights in the world. He always had a very content, happy expression no matter what he was doing—but when that expression spread into a smile, his whole face lit up. His eyes grew, and eyebrows rose, and his teeth appeared, and it was impossible not to smile back at him. He felt it, too. We had found our home.

We stayed there for two more hours: we called our best friends who had lived in the area for a decade to check it out. Another of our best friends from New York, an architect, also happened to be in town and was just five minutes away, so he dropped by, too, to check out the "bones of the house," as he called it. Everyone loved it.

As we walked out of the house, Nick began to explain the significance of this particular street in Laurel Canyon. Jim Morrison had lived in a house on the corner of this street, and it was where he had written his famous song "Love Street." As a tribute, the city had lovingly re-named the street "Love Street" and commemorated it with a little sign at the end of the block.

Our friend Molly, whom Nick called "the mayor of the Canyon" be-cause she knew everyone and everything, was with us. She's fun, vibrant, happy, and hilarious. Molly and her husband, Trevor, know everyone in the Canyon; they know all the fun history and always host the best events at their home. Their home is the most eclectic Canyon "village." I say "village" because surrounding their main house is a small guest-house, a bomb shelter, a tree house, and the coolest man-made bar you'll ever see. Trevor is a film director and experience designer and Molly is a graphic designer. They are Californians to the bone, and, more specif-ically, Laurel Canyonites to the bone.

As we stood there with Molly, she insisted we stop and take a photo in front of the house.

"That's your house, I can feel it," she said. We were going to hang the picture in the living room.

We listened to the song on the drive back up Lookout Mountain. "She lives on Love Street," it began . . . I have a tattoo of the word "love" on my left wrist, and the name Amanda means "worthy of love." It was the last affirmation I needed; I knew it was meant to be. I was getting excited now, too.

I'd seen Nick work tirelessly on two things in his life: creating his one-man show and getting us this house. We had to act fast.

I was filming fitness videos all day for the next three days, so I couldn't help with anything. Anna arrived the following day from New York. At the height of my depression, I had begged her to come out and stay with us—hoping I could ultimately convince her to move to the West Coast. Nick had always said, "If you and Anna go, everyone else will follow."

The three of us headed out to a lofty space downtown where I was filming. I got to work; Anna strapped Elvis to herself and paced around the room, trying to get him to nap; and Nick set to work in the corner.

He did it all—spent the day making phone calls to the bank to secure a loan, asking friends to write reference letters, and preparing a heartfelt essay to the current owners about why we wanted, *needed*, to buy this home. I found this determination so attractive and endearing, it made me excited for the first time about the possibility of his dream becoming our reality. I started to imagine it all: the memories we would make in each room, the holidays we would spend there, the meals we would have around the table. I started to want it for us, too, but I honestly felt that it was not going to happen.

The realtor told us there was a full-cash offer on the table already, with others pending. We couldn't go above the asking price—it was already our maximum budget—and we certainly couldn't offer cash. My sister and I exchanged glances from across the room, communicating in our own wordless language that no one else could ever begin to understand. Nick was in the corner, feverishly shuffling papers, flipping his hair around, and pacing the room on calls. He would hang up, clap his hands together, clench his fists in the victory position, and then move on to the next task on his list. We watched him with a mix of admiration and pity. Anna met my gaze; we both smiled and shook our heads, saying, "Poor guy, he doesn't have a chance at getting that house!"

Two days after we submitted our offer, the phone rang during the middle of breakfast. I was still wet from the shower and nursing Elvis, and Nick was still in his PJs—his hair wild and unruly.

"They are countering our offer—and *only* our offer!" he shouted.

"They loved our application and want us to have the first right of refusal. We got the house!" He stood up and swept Elvis and me into a huge hug.

"Elvito, we got you a house!"

Anna snapped a photo of us without us knowing it, and our expressions say it all.

I was in disbelief.

Anna was in disbelief.

Nick was thrilled.

We were going to be homeowners in Laurel Canyon.

I couldn't help but be excited, too. I had spent twenty years living in tiny apartments in New York. I wasn't ready to leave, but I had always wanted a home. Now we had one, and it felt right.

To complete the serendipitous chain of events, the next day was the famous Laurel Canyon Photo Day. It's a tradition in the neighborhood going back decades; all the current residents of the Canyon gather in front of the Canyon Country Store to take a big group photo. Photographs hang in the store and show how the community has grown and changed over the years.

There's live music and mingling, and everyone arrives in their full Canyon glory: flannels and long wavy hair and costumes and guitars. If you didn't know, you would think you were at a reenactment of Woodstock. Anna and I went down early to get coffees at Lily's, and Nick was going to come later. As we arrived, we saw a band set up, playing an impromptu concert in the parking lot. I turned to Anna and said, "How much you want to bet that next year, Nick is in that band, playing on Photo Day."

I saw him walking down the hill from at least a hundred feet away, in a Canadian tuxedo: dark jeans and a chambray button-down shirt. He wore his father's medallion and other gold jewelry on his wrists and fingers. The look was finished with sunglasses; long, dark, wavy hair; and a glowing smile. He was right where he was meant to be.

A chant began after the photo was snapped. Everyone chanting in unison,

"We are Laurel Canyon!"

"We are Laurel Canyon!"

"We are Laurel Canyon!"

I was crying. I looked over and saw Anna was crying, too.

She told me later how special it had been to witness that moment: Nick and me on day one of our new chapter, in this wonderful new community, with a charming new house and our beautiful baby boy. It really felt like the start of something special.

I looked up at Nick and kissed him after the last round of the chant. I knew we had done the right thing.

In March, our lease was finally over. We had to go back to Manhattan to pack up and officially move everything.

I've gone back and wondered a million times when or where Nick got COVID, but I'll never know. It might have been on the plane; it might have been in New York . . . I guess it doesn't matter. Still, it's impossible not to wonder—what if we'd never gone back for our stuff? Nick had even proposed the idea of just letting the movers handle everything for us, go in and pack up and drive it here for us to sort. But that felt impossible. There was too much to sort through. My family was there, eagerly awaiting a visit. Anna had moved to Paris that January and was flying back to New York to see us. I had a week of classes and privates already scheduled in New York, from which we badly needed the income.

In March, COVID was in the news and growing more severe every day, but the hysteria had yet to hit the United States and seemed to be a bit overhyped to both of us. It was the early days of this virus, when so much was still unknown, and we said to each other, "We're young; even if we were to get it, we would be okay."

We flew separately because *Rock of Ages* had opened, so Nick was working, and I wanted the extra time with my family. Nick had not been back to New York since we left the past September. The day he arrived, he immediately performed at a charity concert on Forty-Second Street. He took the red-eye, went right into a rehearsal, came home to shower for a minute, then went back out to perform. When he finally got home that night, he was exhausted.

It felt comforting to be back in New York, back to packed classes, and back with my family. It was March 9, the depths of New York's coldest temperatures. I spent the week riding the subway around Manhattan, running to and from my classes, and working on the apartment at night. After Nick performed, he got to work on the apartment, spending the entire day packing and sorting and donating. We barely saw each other during the day, and he didn't like that I was out and about in the city, teaching classes as things got worse.

For the first days of our trip, New York felt entirely normal. COVID was all over the news, but it felt distant. It was mostly reports from Italy and China, and life in New York was still the same.

But that didn't last long. By March 12, businesses were closing left and right, and fewer people were on the street. The subway was almost empty, as were the shelves at the grocery stores. I was still teaching my fitness classes because gyms were not closed. People could keep enough distance from one another in the studio, and my classes required no equipment. I didn't touch anyone or anything, so I felt very secure. I questioned the safety of riding the subway, but it was almost abandoned. Each night, my family gathered for dinner at my parents' apartment. My sister Alison and my niece were just a few blocks away and would walk down to join us. We cooked in to avoid being out, and we watched the news, wondering how worried we needed to be. My brother, Todd, and his family were safe in San Francisco. My oldest sister, Traci, and her family had already been isolated for several weeks in Houston. Anna was still in France. Her flight back to the United States had been canceled, and she was too afraid to rebook it, though we urged her to try to get back.

"I've been living here for the last eight weeks; I must have been exposed," she said. "It's too dangerous for me to come back and be with you all. I have to stay here two weeks and ensure I have no symptoms before I can think about flying back. I'll be okay if I get it—I'm young, I'm healthy. We need to protect Mom and Dad."

She called from Paris on March 15. The city was going into lockdown with no warning. Two days before, everything had been normal, and suddenly there had been a considerable spike in cases overnight. Every restaurant, school, and business had been ordered to close. It was midnight there, this had just been announced, and she was hysterical and terrified.

"This will happen in America, too," she warned us. "The virus is spreading—do not leave the apartment for any reason, and please do not leave each other."

We thought she was overreacting. We had seen the stories from Europe on the news. "It's not like that here," we told her. "Everyone is being safe and respectful. New York is fine." New York still felt fine.

But by that weekend, more of the city had shut down, and it really started to feel eerie. New York is such a bustling, chaotic city, and it had fallen silent. Streets were empty, stores were boarded up, and traffic was nonexistent. The only sound was an occasional ambulance buzzing down the street, and the frequency of them grew steadily. Nick and I started to question whether it was safe to fly back to Los Angeles.

As we watched the news every night, the world was getting scarier and scarier. Cases were rising, but no one really knew what that meant, what would happen next, and how long this would last. Stores were entirely out of hand sanitizer, soap, gloves, and toilet paper. You could not buy a mask anywhere. Anna called us in tears nightly, adding to my fear. Europe was ahead of the United States in numbers. She was already living with the reality that wouldn't fully hit us for another two weeks, and trying to weigh the danger of flying back to America. We urged her to come home, and she begged us all to drive to Ohio together, where my parents still had their house. Leave New York, forget about LA right now, and get somewhere safe, stay together. She eventually decided to fly back to Ohio ten days later on March 25. She was terrified to fly, but said she had a gut feeling that she needed to come home.

We sat in our empty apartment on March 16, in utter confusion and fear, as the movers were carrying the final boxes out. We had three choices: stay in New York with my parents, go to Ohio all together, or fly back to Los Angeles. All of our things had just been packed onto a truck and would be arriving in LA in only two weeks. Our home was being renovated; there were daily decisions to make and things to oversee. Nick and I fought and talked in circles about what to do. He wanted to go; I wanted to stay. We weren't even sure our flight would take off—they were being canceled left and right, as travel was deemed dangerous and discouraged unless it was absolutely necessary.

The night before we were supposed to fly, I was sleeping on my parents' couch, and Nick was on a blow-up mattress on the floor. I was sobbing and terrified of making the wrong choice.

"What are we going to do, Amanda?" he said.

And I just kept saying, "I don't know. I don't know what we should do."

On the morning of our flight, we stood together on the street, saying goodbye to my parents. We all had tears streaming down our faces. I have seen my dad cry only a few times in my life, and it scared me to death how hard he cried as he hugged Nick. The last thing he said to him was "Take care of your family."

The words replayed in my head as we drove away from New York.

What if my parents got sick? What if they needed us? What if we needed them?

It felt so final, this taxi ride, this goodbye. I had the strangest feeling it would be a very long time before we would see New York again.

As the city quickly passed by and slowly faded out of sight, I thought about all the memories we have in New York. Not the big ones, but the little ones. The ones I knew were most at risk of being forgotten as time went on. Enjoying all of our picnics and walks in Central Park. Strolling around the Upper West Side with our dogs, on the hunt for a Mister Softee ice-cream cone covered in rainbow sprinkles—one of my many pregnancy cravings. Gathering for family dinners with my parents and sisters last summer. Sharing Negronis and lasagna at our favorite restaurant, Cafe Fiorello, at "our" table outside. Walking along the Hudson holding hands and pushing Elvis's stroller.

I thought back to my early days here. Auditions in crowded rooms, and opening nights on Broadway. The first time I did an eye-high kick on the stage at Radio City. Late nights at the hidden speakeasy on Forty-Sixth Street, followed by grilled-cheese sandwiches and milk-shakes at a twenty-four-hour diner. Taking my goddaughter to the American Museum of Natural History, meeting my sister for impromptu manicures, or smoothies, or Sunday-evening church. Lugging my life around Manhattan in various tote bags—always ready for whatever the day could throw at me. Watching the Thanksgiving Day Parade, and standing in line for the Shake Shack, and walking down Fifth Avenue at Christmastime to see the windows and the lights.

I had hoped I'd be calm by the time we reached JFK, but I only felt worse. We called Nick's mom, Lesley, in tears, looking for direction.

"You have a home now in Los Angeles," she said. "You have all your stuff on a truck arriving in LA in two weeks. You are doing the right thing."

It calmed us. She was right. If we went to Ohio, we didn't know when or even if we could get back to Los Angeles. They could shut down flights at any moment. There was too much uncertainty. Everyone was being told to go home and stay home. LA was our home now.

We were through security and at our gate in minutes. JFK was empty, spooky. No one was flying, which was both scary and comforting.

We had upgraded ourselves to first class to have extra distance from people. We wiped everything down and were careful not to touch anything. We wore masks and gloves, and we felt safe.

"Honey, I think we're doing the right thing," Nick said once we had settled. And I agreed.

We made it back to California. We felt so safe. We had successfully packed up our life, moved everything, said our goodbyes, and flown cross-country during a pandemic. The scary part was finally over. *We are going to be okay*, we thought.

Now I look back and think we should never have gone to New York.

three

I always look for the silver linings in hard times, and the silver lining of having a baby during this crisis was that he ultimately saved me. Elvis kept me from curling up into a ball and sobbing all day. There isn't the option of moping around or staying in bed when you have a child to care for. You are forced to wake up, be present, play, smile, and entertain the little person who is counting on you for everything. Elvis made me start each day happy, forced me to laugh, and allowed me to think about something other than how scared I was. I didn't have my husband at home, but I had our son.

After I shared my story on Instagram, people worldwide—from Boston to Bangkok—started praying for Nick. All the love and support that was coming my way helped me feel like I wasn't alone, and the innate kindness of people during a pandemic continued to amaze me. I'm not sure the response would have been the same had we not been in the middle of a forced lockdown. With the world on pause, everyone had time for each other once again, time to listen. Friends close to me could imagine themselves in my shoes, but people I had never met could, too. Whether they knew us or not, they truly cared.

The first two weeks of April felt like the most threatening of the whole spring since so much was unknown. People were still processing what was going on, and everything about life had changed so fast in March that it seemed as if anything could happen next. We weren't yet sure about how the virus spread—we only knew it was happening, and happening fast. It seemed that if you went anywhere, saw anyone, did anything—you would get the virus. It was on the news that cases were expected to peak soon, and every TV channel, radio station, and newspaper was reporting the same message: *"Do not leave your home!"* People wanted to come help me, but with what had happened to Nick, I was on high alert. If Nick tested positive, then there was a chance COVID was still lurking on the surfaces of our house, or that I was also infected and not yet showing symptoms. So I passed the first ten days of this journey home alone with Elvis.

I started off each morning with an AK! Positive Thought of the Day. I had been doing this on my Instagram stories for the last three years. I'd share a thought or a quote that would keep me focused and set me up to have an optimistic day. Now more than ever, I needed them. So on day one, I chose a quote by Fred Rogers: "Look for the helpers. You will always find people who are helping." It was precisely how I felt.

When I look back now on the help I received, I can only see God behind all of it. Every day I prayed for a miracle, and every day miracles appeared in the form of generosity from complete strangers all over the world. People gave me their time, money, advice, encouragement, resources, and love. They weren't just giving these things to me but, in the end, to my whole family. They were doing it out of the pure kindness of their hearts.

That week alone, Matt Weaver, the producer of *Rock of Ages*, continued to take care of all my groceries, texting me every time he went to Whole Foods to ask me what I needed. The owner of Bandier and my friend Michelle stepped in to provide meals for Elvis. Weekly deliveries of gourmet, organic baby food arrived for him, so I never had to worry about what he would eat.

Chandra, a new client of mine in LA, reached out right away, asking how she could help. She started by sending a dinner and a neck massager to me, and her kind gestures never stopped.

One of my friends, Vasthy, from *Good Vibrations*, my first Broadway show, had also just moved to LA, and she offered to come by that afternoon to play a music class for Elvis from behind the screen door.

"E-L-V-I-S—Elvis is my name," she sang. Broadway people are the most incredible and inspiring people to me. Even brand-new friends I had just made in LA were leaving things in my driveway: groceries, coffee, face masks, bath salts, toys for Elvis, and bouquets of flowers. Everyone was just trying to help ease and brighten my day.

I have always believed that people are innately good, and that we should ask for help when we need it and accept help when it's offered. I saw the real power of this when I first started my own business. I knew I couldn't do it all alone, and I didn't have all the answers. I couldn't have done this alone either. I didn't let pride or fear get in the way of accepting everything that was offered to me, because I was desperate for answers, aid, and advice. I saw each act of kindness as an act of God. People would message me daily, saying, "I've never prayed in my life, and I just got down on my knees and prayed for your family." I asked God over and over again for my miracle, but I always prayed, "Your will be done." I believe God showed himself and his goodness to me, to my family, and to the whole world through the help I received throughout this fight.

"Musical Morning" with Elvis is another routine of mine. I play a song each morning and capture Elvis doing whatever cute, naughty, or mundane thing he's doing at that moment, then share it on Instagram. I had been doing that since he was just a few days old, and in a way, it's now like a virtual baby book set to music. This day, and every day that first week, I picked a song that Nick loved and dedicated it to him. I played Prince's "Purple Rain" that first morning because Nick loved it and sang it any time he could—benefit concert or karaoke night, he loved singing "Purple Rain." Nick always told a story about one of the times he saw him in concert. Prince asked the audience, "Is it better to give or receive?" He offered the microphone to someone in the front row, and the guy said, "Give." Prince said, "Then give that man in the back row your front-row seat. You don't tell Prince no," and so the guy did it! Prince then asked someone else, and she said, "Receive." Prince offered the woman his hand and pulled her onto the stage, then sang "Purple Rain" to her. The whole audience went crazy.

I continued my daily videos of Elvis for Nick. I think sending them helped me feel normal, like maybe he was just away on a trip and not in the hospital in a coma. I thought about how I would feel if I had missed ten days of our baby's life. Elvis changed every single day; I didn't want Nick to miss a minute of it. Distanced "visits" from my neighbors continued and gave me something to do. Elvis's Stroller Buddies now came twice each day to take him around Laurel Canyon so I could have two hours alone to get something done. I usually spent them working on my business as my fear of the growing hospital bills mounted.

I launched my subscription series right as quarantine began. I'd been a fitness instructor for four years but had only taught live at studios, except for a few videos I did for my own website when it first launched. Those had been such a production to film; it was weeks of choosing the right music, outfits, backgrounds, and routines to look polished and perfect. I flew to LA to film with my whole team. I watched my diet for days ahead of time so that my body would look toned, and I had a hair and makeup team touching me up throughout. My videos did well on my website, and people told me they enjoyed taking my classes from their homes. So I had wanted to do some kind of app or streaming service for a while, but matching that level of perfection postponed it. But this time around, I didn't have the time or money to do it. On top of that, I had the new full-time job of being a mom. I was breastfeeding and caring for Elvis, in addition to teaching at Studio B, getting settled in LA, and starting the renovations of the house. I thought no one would subscribe if it was just me in my driveway, filming on an iPhone. My ideals were holding me back from moving forward.

But quarantine took the expectation of perfection and threw it out the window. Everyone lost their ability to do things the exact way that they wanted. No one's job could go on as it had previously. We got to bend the rules; we got to experiment and see what we could create under the new limitations. And since everyone was in the same boat, everyone was understanding. Perfection wasn't required anymore. In fact, it was annoying to see as everyone's life was in chaos.

I had been training Aimee Song, a famous fashion blogger, on and off for four years. She lived in LA but would often travel, and when we were in the same city, we'd meet for a session. I loved training Aimee. She's a smart woman who built her business from the ground up, full of positive energy, kind, and, most of all, genuine. I offered to train her via Zoom, but she suggested we take the workouts live and share them on Instagram. With all the gyms and studios across the country closed, everyone was forced to get creative with their daily regimens. Skipping workouts was a lot harder to justify while you were at home with absolutely nowhere to go and nothing else to do. I loved the idea as soon as she said it. I knew how difficult this time was for people; they were losing jobs, worried about money, and living in fear of even going outside. I've always found exercise therapeutic, a way to release stress and anxiety. It is a reason to get dressed, and put on uplifting, loud music, and move your body around and work hard at something. I always feel better at the end of a workout. I loved the idea of helping to bring a little happiness into someone's home during this awful time. It was also something to look forward to and a way to talk and connect to other people.

When the news came the night before that Nick was going on the ventilator, I almost canceled the workout we had scheduled, but I knew that I'd have company if I did it. With Aimee and everyone joining in, I'd have an army, support, and love. So I filled her in and said, "I need you today to be my trainer in a sense."

When the private health-care team called to give me an update from the hospital, I always asked if I could visit. But the answer was always no. It broke my heart, but I understood. Nick was sleeping and, by all accounts, seemed to be doing well. Dr. Ng said to me from day one: "Amanda, this is a marathon, not a sprint." He told me most patients are on the vent for fourteen to seventeen days and to remain positive. "If we stay positive, we have options," he always said.

I didn't understand a lot of what the daily updates actually meant during those early days. Hospital jargon is like another language. I think the team knew that I didn't know what anything meant, so they provided an elementary explanation for me, telling me things like, "He did okay overnight. His blood pressure dipped a little, so we had to start him on some medications. The oxygen saturation rate looks good. His vent settings are slowly coming down, so once we get that in a good place, we can talk about getting him off of it."

I didn't ask many questions. I honestly didn't know that I could; this whole process was so new to me. It seemed as though he was improving, and things were slowly getting better, and it was usually a very calm and optimistic phone call. I was naive and new to this world of hospitals and doctors, and critical care. I didn't know what the procedures were, and I didn't know what I was entitled to ask, do, or know as his wife. The rules put in place by COVID created a detachment from it all for me, and I imagine those rules did the same for many families.

Being removed from the hospital entirely that first week kept me from understanding the gravity of the situation. When you aren't there witnessing it, it's harder to believe that it's even happening. I knew Nick was in the ICU, in a coma. But that's all I knew. I didn't yet know how sad and dark the room looked, how cold it was, how quiet it was in there with him asleep and no television or radio on. I couldn't see the tubes connecting his body to the ventilator or the towers they connected to, to keep him breathing. I couldn't see any of that; I could just listen to positive phone calls and take away from them the message, "He is improving."

I continued having nightly FaceTimes with Anna while I ate my dinner, so I didn't feel like I was alone in the evening. She was still alone in quarantine in Ohio, so she looked forward to them, too. I'd update her on what the doctors told me, and then we'd talk about nothing for an hour. It felt so good just to laugh, to be silly, to talk nonsense. Every night we talked about how we wished she could come out and be with me. But she still had another week to spend in quarantine before she was sure she had no symptoms.

"When my two weeks are up," she said, "I'll get on the first flight there—if I'm allowed."

She looked up one-way flights from Canton to Los Angeles, just to see if there were options. That flight would typically cost around $500 if booked far enough in advance. But because of COVID and the fact that no one was flying, it was only $26!

I asked the doctors the next day when I spoke with them, but they said no. Travel was dangerous, I was potentially dangerous, and exposure to anyone was dangerous. Dr. Ng told me no one should come unless I really, really needed the help.

Talking to family at night helped me not to feel alone. I was so thankful that we were so close and that I had such a good relationship with Nick's mom and siblings, too. With everything else gone—work, parties, parks, events—people were all we had during lockdown. It was a time to stop and realize that fact: that when everything else is taken away, all you have are the ones you love and who love you back. I had a lot of love, and I had my faith.

I've always found comfort in the poem "Footprints in the Sand," about how, during the most challenging moments in your life, when you feel alone, God isn't just there with you, he's actually carrying you. My faith has always been important to me, but that week I was so grateful to have it. Knowing God was in control got me through the hardest times. I knew I was in his hands, and he was carrying Nick and me. Midweek, Dr. Ng said Nick was making good progress, and with a couple more days like this—they would be able to take him off the ventilator! This was the first sign of a light at the end of the tunnel. There wasn't a bone in my body that didn't believe that he was coming home soon.

With everything else going on, our moving truck arrived from New York and was supposed to be unpacked into our new home. But our house was far from ready. With Nick now in the ICU, I was desperately trying to figure out what to do with our things. I had no idea where to put everything, so I called a storage facility to rent a unit. We still had many decisions that needed to be made about our home. I was going to the new house to check on the construction and make choices without Nick. I hated doing all this on my own. It was his dream house, and he was missing out, unable to be a part of it.

The update from the team on the night of April 3 was that Nick's third and final test came back positive. We finally had a definitive answer. It was scary to think two tests had been negative. How many other people received negative tests when they were actually positive in those early days?

With this confirmation, private health sent a nurse to the house that evening to give me a COVID test. I had no symptoms, but they wanted to make sure. At that time, getting tested was a privilege, and I felt lucky. The nurse arrived in full PPE, and I stood in the driveway to get my nose swabbed. The nurse stuck a long cotton swab up each nostril, wiggling it around to scrape the inside of my nose. It caused my eyes to tear up, and felt as if I had just ingested seawater.

They also started proning Nick, a technique where they turn the patient onto his belly to open the lungs. This position allows the lungs to expand, improving oxygenation. Hospitals around the world were doing this to help COVID patients breathe. It seems like the position would actually make it harder to breathe, but it has the reverse effect. Nick's body responded well to the proning, and it was yet another reason to believe he was recovering.

As I awaited my test results, I knew I needed to come up with a plan for Elvis in case something happened to me. Nick was in a coma, my parents were on the other side of the country, and Nick's family was in Toronto. I realized I had nothing in place in the event of a catastrophe. No living will, no plan for who would get custody of Elvis. Nick and I had talked about setting up a will, and a trust, especially after buying our first home. But we never followed through. There's no excuse; it's just something you think you won't need to do until you're older, so, with everything else going on around us, we put it off. Now it was vital, and I had nothing. My dad had been telling me to do it since the day Elvis was born.

"I know, Dad, I'll get to it," I always replied.

He was also on us repeatedly about taking out life insurance. He was an insurance salesman, and he was not going to let this one go. He hounded me daily through emails, texts, and calls. "Did you get the policy yet, Amanda?"

I got so annoyed that I finally followed through on it just before we left New York, so we had life insurance in case anything happened to one of us. I would have never done that without my dad. Parents always know best.

But we hadn't gotten around to writing our wills. So I called my friend Rachel and started to cry as I tried to get the words out. "If anything were to happen to me right now, would you and Rickey be able to take care of Elvis until my family can get here?" She said, "Of course," and I felt some small relief knowing that at least I had something in place for Elvis. He was the most precious thing in the world.

I have always wanted to be a mom, and Nick always wanted to be a dad. It was one of the things I loved about him. I was a little nervous about being able to conceive because I had been told by two doctors that my egg count was low. "You should have tried five years ago" was a direct quote from one doctor after seeing the results of my blood tests. It crushed me. I'd heard so many stories from women who have difficulty getting pregnant—I knew it could be a long road. I was already thirty-six; my chances were just getting slimmer. A few of my close girlfriends already had babies, and my sister had just gotten pregnant. I had terrible baby fever, and I was prepared to do whatever it took to be a mom.

Nick and I decided that we would try on our own first, just to see what happened, despite my bad egg count. We were in New Orleans for his fortieth birthday. We wanted to do something special to celebrate, and it was a city he had never been to, one known for its music. We planned to spend the weekend going to jazz clubs, and eating Creole food, and staying awake dancing until late into the night.

I booked a hotel on Bourbon Street because I thought we needed to be right in the action. I should have known better after living in New York City for nineteen years. It's like telling someone to book a hotel on Forty-Second Street in Times Square! We arrived on a Tuesday, and the bars around the hotel were packed with adults acting like they had just turned twenty-one. We had to laugh; it was New Orleans, after all. I had paid for a suite, so I was disappointed to walk into our hotel room and find that it smelled like alcohol and had holes in the walls, dirty carpet, and cracks in the bathtub! "This simply won't do," I said. "It's your fortieth!" Nick hated complaining about these types of things, but I had paid for a special room, and this wasn't going to cut it. They showed us another room, right on the street. It was in slightly better condition but opened right on Bourbon Street, and even at three p.m. it was already loud, so we knew that by midnight we would have no chance of sleeping. The third room finally fit the bill. It was on the newer, renovated side, away from the street, and larger. I was happy; the third time's a charm!

I was ovulating that weekend, so it seemed the perfect time to try. It was our second planned attempt. The first had been a couple months prior on our honeymoon. Nick kept saying, "You spend your whole life trying to keep the sperm away, and then it's so hard to get them in when you finally want to!" A couple weeks later, I just had a feeling. The only test I had at home was one I'd bought in Italy on our honeymoon, so I went to the bathroom first thing in the morning to see.

Positive. I was shocked! Two times and it worked? I'd thought I didn't have any eggs, and it would be a very long process. It felt like the biggest blessing in the world.

I ran out to find Nick, who had the dogs ready to go for a morning walk in Central Park. I said, "Oh my God, Nick, we are pregnant!"

But I wasn't totally sure we could trust this test. It was Italian and a couple months old. I wasn't sure why, but I felt like maybe it was faulty.

"Can you run to Duane Reade and buy another test?" I asked him.

His exact words were "I'll go take the dogs to the park, and bring them back, and then go to the store."

I said, "What? *No!* We could be pregnant, go *now!*"

Three positive tests later, we were both convinced that we were having a baby.

Elvis was conceived on Nick's fortieth birthday, in New Orleans, on Bourbon Street.

"This kid will have music in his bones!" Nick said.

I had to rush off to teach a private client, and I skipped up Central Park West to get to her apartment. I had wanted to be a mom my whole life, and now I was lucky enough to be pregnant. I thanked God the entire way there and every day after.

Two days after my COVID test, I got a phone call from the private health-care team, and they told me that it came back negative. I was shocked. I thought for sure that I had it and was just asymptomatic. A million questions arose in my mind, but mainly—how did Nick get it and I didn't? I asked Dr. Ng, and he said there was no rhyme or reason. He said sometimes whole families got the virus, and sometimes just one person in the entire household. I tested for antibodies not long after and did not have them either. It didn't make any sense, but I was just thankful to be healthy.

The hospital also told me on that call about a new medical trial that they thought Nick should be a part of. He fit all the criteria to be a candidate, but they needed my consent to start it. It was for a drug called remdesivir. There were two groups: one that would receive a placebo and one that would get the drug for three days. I would never know which group Nick would be in, but they believed that this drug would help COVID symptoms, so it seemed like there was nothing to lose. I had no idea what this drug was, nor did I know anything about medical trials. I did a quick search, and I called a family friend who is an expert in the medical field. Before I could even finish explaining what I knew of the trial to him, he said, "I know exactly what you're talking about, Amanda. Do it now!"

I hung up the phone, called Dr. Ng back, and said, "Let's do it."

This was the first time they called me "to get my consent," the first of many times I had to give the okay on something that could potentially change the course of Nick's life. I didn't know at this point that they called to ask your opinion, let alone get approval, or that I would have to make several significant decisions over the next months. Every time they called me to ask for my consent, my stomach dropped. I always trusted the doctor's opinion and wanted to do what the medical team felt was best, but having to be the one to make that choice every time was scary.

I could barely pronounce remdesivir when I was trying to repeat it five minutes later to Nick's mom. She fully trusted me as Nick's wife to make the final call, but I tried to talk everything through with her. Lesley had been in the hospital with Nick's father just three years before, so she could put herself in my shoes and speak from experience. Since this was a medical trial, we will never know for sure if Nick received the drug, but based on how Nick's body was responding those first ten days, it seemed that he did get it, and that it did help him.

The other call that came from the hospital that week was from Debra, a social worker who had been assigned to my case. She called and introduced herself in a hushed, sad tone, asking me how I was doing and what she could do for me. I remember thinking it was so strange.

Why did she call? I wondered.

It was nice, I thought, *but why do I need a social worker? What would she help me with?*

I did not yet fully grasp all that comes along with having a loved one in the ICU—the emotions, the stress, the anxiety. A social worker is assigned to the case to help the patient's family cope with all of this. But I wasn't really going through anything just yet. It was all new at that stage. I would later learn all the ropes and how to climb them. But at that point, I was trying to get through the day as a single mom.

I had never been alone with Elvis for that long of a period, nor confined to such a small space with him. He was nine months old and into everything. He moved around the floor in a one-legged crab-style crawl, and trouble followed him wherever he went. He got into the kitchen cabinets and pulled out cleaning supplies, heavy serving dishes, and appliances that I had tried to tuck away. He loved to crawl into the spare closet and go for the cast-iron fire poker, which I had tried my best to hide but he always seemed to find. The whole house was suddenly a threat. I couldn't install safety things or remove anything from the walls because it wasn't my house. I tried to keep all the doors to other rooms closed and taped the cabinets shut. "That's a no thank you," I said to him when he did something naughty, but it didn't help. The only time I could really relax was if he was sleeping or out on a walk.

That night was the first night of an outdoor concert series that our neighbor Jono had started from his roof; it was called "Music in the Canyon." There wasn't much you could do to help people during those weeks, but Jono had this beautiful idea that was so perfect for this community. Elvis and I walked outside and joined Molly and Trevor to listen along with the rest of the neighborhood. We sat six feet away from each other, yet we were so close in mind, body, and spirit as we listened.

It was something to do, a reason to get out of the house and escape my reality for a few minutes. It also gave me people to be with, and the music made me feel close to Nick. Jono was hosting some new musicians from Ireland at the time. The lead singer, Lenii, wore two long French braids, played the piano, and sang her songs in a very haunting, husky, alto voice. It was beautiful. They sang "Falling Slowly" that night.

Raise your hopeful voice, you have a choice
You'll make it now

I enjoyed it, but I cried as they played. I felt so lonely and over-whelmed with my entire situation. These impromptu concerts are why Nick wanted to live here. I wished he was with me. It wasn't fair, all that he was missing.

I downloaded the TikTok app later that night and became addicted to how distracting it was, how it could kill hours in what felt like minutes. I decided to start learning some of the dances. It took me a whole night to nail J.Lo's Super Bowl dance, but it was fun. I watched TV some nights. I got sucked into *Tiger King*, like the rest of America. Anything to take my mind off the hospital was good, even if it was just for an hour.

Some nights I'd pass out on the couch at nine, and others I'd still be wide-eyed at two in the morning. My mind would wander, and I'd imagine my poor husband there alone, sedated, ten minutes down the street. There was nothing I wanted to do more than run there, grab him, and bring him home. It hurt so much that I couldn't do anything about it, and he had no idea what was going on, either in the world at large or in our own little world. Neither did Elvis—he was a baby. I knew one day he would have questions about this. He would want to hear the stories and understand everything. I wanted to make sure that I remembered how I was feeling and what we were doing every day. We had become buddies through this, and I wanted to document it all for him, too. It felt important because of how unprecedented this time was. When I couldn't sleep, one night, I got out a piece of paper and decided to write Elvis a letter. When I was done, I finally managed to drift off to sleep.

The next morning was Palm Sunday. It felt so strange not to be going to church. Nick was having a great day, according to the doctors. His body was responding well to the medications, and they told me in a couple more days, he would be off the vent. I was so happy I called Nick's mom and my parents to tell them, almost unable to get the words out through my tears. At this rate, he would be home next week.

Despite that light at the end of the tunnel, being alone with Elvis was starting to wear me down. I had two breakdowns that morning. I think he could sense my anxiety, and he became extra clingy. I couldn't put him down without him screaming. But I had so much to do: make new workout videos, keep the house clean, manage the crazy amount of emails and text messages I received, and take in all the deliveries.

At that time, people thought COVID lingered on surfaces. So the daily tower of boxes that arrived had to be disinfected before they could be opened, broken down, and put into the recycling. When flowers arrived, the box needed to be sanitized, then the flowers cut and put into water. I didn't have enough vases to display them all. Everything was sent with such good intentions, but managing everything was becoming overwhelming.

When Elvis went down for a nap that day, I realized how much I just missed my husband. I missed seeing him walk through the door. I missed his voice and smile. I missed seeing him with Elvis. I looked through photos on my phone of them together. I cherish every photo I ever took now and wish I had a thousand more. I had reached a low point. That evening Molly and Trevor called me and told me to come to the driveway. As I came out of the house, a truck arrived with Jono, Lenii, and the other musicians that Jono was hosting. From the street, they played "You've Got a Friend" for me, and I sat with Elvis in my lap on the stairs to my front door and let all the tears I had been holding in come out. I couldn't wait to tell Nick about all of this once he was back. He would be so proud of his neighborhood. As I fell asleep that night, I thought about all the health heroes in the world, and especially the team of people helping Nick. They, too, were missing things happening in their families. They also had spouses and babies and extended families. They worked tirelessly from day to night to save other people's lives while putting their own lives in danger. I felt so thankful for them all, and so amazed by their sacrifice.

I woke up to a rare, rainy day in LA, and the gloomy sky did not help my mood. But I tried to fill the day with fun activities for Elvis and me. I needed to get in a workout, but he needed to be entertained. So I pulled out old dances and songs and performed for him. I wheeled his baby activity center, which I called his "office," into the bathroom so I could shower, dry my hair, and get dressed, all while singing "Wheels on the Bus." Then I decided to really put on a show and film it for Nick as my video of the day. I knew he would appreciate my Broadway efforts for Elvis. I did excerpts from *42nd Street*, Rockette dance numbers, and *Bullets over Broadway* while Elvis looked on, utterly unimpressed. He did the best deadpan to the camera during one video, as if he was telling Nick, "Dada, please get home fast. Mom is losing it!"

Nick came off the hydroxychloroquine that day, and we were waiting for his body to require zero assistance on breathing so they could take him off the vent. "It should be any day now," the doctors told me. Everything was looking positive. We were almost there. It had been such a tough week, but it was almost over. But a call the morning of April 10 changed everything. I could tell something was off from the moment Dr. Ng started talking.

"It was a rough night. Nick got an infection, which caused him to suddenly spike a fever, and then his blood pressure to drop . . .

"His heart stopped, Amanda. He died for two minutes, coded on the table.

"We were able to resuscitate him, but I'll be honest with you: right now, his survival is minute to minute . . ."

four

He died for two minutes.

He *died* for two minutes?

He died for two minutes?!

That phone call was the first time I was hit with the reality that I could lose my husband to COVID. That phone call changed my life forever.

I burst into tears but tried to keep it together enough to finish the conversation. My stomach felt nauseous, and chills came over me. Dr. Ng continued to explain what was happening. Nick was in a critical state, but somewhat stable, and they were taking him into emergency surgery to save his life.

The only way to keep Nick alive now was to put him on ECMO, a machine that essentially keeps your heart and lungs functioning for you until you're strong enough to do it yourself. He told me this in such a calm, collected tone that I didn't really understand the severity of what he was saying. An ECMO machine is a last-ditch effort, a machine you go on only if you are *seriously ill*. I didn't know this at the time; I had never heard of an ECMO before. The only thing I kept hearing and replaying in my head were the words "He died for two minutes."

Dr. Ng told me the hospital was going to call me as soon as we hung up to get my consent, and Dr. Williams, who would be performing the surgery, would explain to me what would happen. I had never spoken directly to the hospital. I honestly hadn't realized that I could. Dr. Williams explained the surgery would be to put four cannulas into Nick to connect him to the ECMO machine. Some hospitals didn't have this machine at all, so we were lucky that Cedars had one available or else Nick would have died right then and there. It was not a simple surgery, and there was a possibility that he wouldn't survive. His body was already in a fragile condition, and there is always a risk of complications. He said he would call me back when it was done to let me know if it had been successful. There was nothing I could do but to sit and wait.

I'm so grateful that Elvis was just a baby. That he won't remember that day. He won't remember that I started shaking and fell to the ground. He won't remember that I couldn't breathe, and that I desperately called my friends in the Canyon, trying to get out the words to tell them what was happening. I didn't even know what I was saying; I couldn't explain what the doctors had told me or make any sense of anything. I couldn't even repeat ECMO; I was calling it EXMO.

"He can't die," I sobbed into the phone. "Elvis needs his dad. I need my husband. This can't be happening."

I tried to tell Lesley and my parents, but I wasn't making any sense. None of this made sense to me. My parents, at home with my sisters Ali and Anna on speakerphone, were just as hysterical. This had come out of nowhere. Everyone wanted to understand more, ask more questions, know exactly what happened, but I couldn't help them. I couldn't explain it. Lesley was in shock when I called her. She stayed very calm, but I could hear the fear in her voice. It didn't feel real to me, and I was just down the street from the hospital; Lesley was in another country, thousands of miles away. This couldn't register correctly.

There was nothing I could do. I started praying, asking God for help.

"Lord, please help my husband. Please be with the doctors. Lord, keep him safe and in your care." I repeated it over and over again, on my knees in the kitchen, still by the phone. Elvis was crawling around the floor, getting into things as usual, and seemed completely unaware that anything was off.

Trevor and Molly came rushing down. Molly grabbed Elvis to take him out on a walk right away, and Trevor grabbed me, wrapping me tight into one of his big bear hugs, and we sat there together, crying in the kitchen of Brown Bear.

I couldn't get myself up from the floor; my legs felt too weak to stand on. I went through an entire roll of toilet paper as I blew my nose and wiped away tears. Zach arrived, walking into his own guesthouse for the first time in weeks; he was in shock at the scene. As a director, actor, and screenwriter, he must have felt like he was walking into a scene from a movie. It was that surreal to all of us. None of us knew what to do; there was nothing that could be done. We were all in complete shock. Trevor and Zach had never seen me cry like that. I had never cried like that before.

I remember begging and pleading with God to keep him alive, to let him live for Elvis. They just stared at me, unable to offer any words to comfort me. There was nothing anyone could say at that moment to help me, but just their presence was helpful. It was the first time in weeks we had seen each other up close or hugged each other. COVID rules had to be set aside; it was an emergency. It felt so strange to hug someone again after weeks of hugging not being allowed. Hugs usually make you feel comforted, but during COVID, they made you feel uneasy. Today, they were vital. Without my friends in the neighborhood, without that hug from Trevor—I may not have made it through the day.

My brother called after talking to my parents and learning what happened. He was already packing his bag and was planning to leave the next morning. The six-hour drive meant he would be in LA by early evening. Just to know that family was coming was a huge relief. Todd had just visited a few months before. Elvis loved him, and I knew that a male presence in the house would bring me comfort. My brother is the oldest and had moved to the West Coast fifteen years before. I didn't get to spend much time with him over the past few years, but we are incredibly close nonetheless. It meant the world to me that he was coming.

When I moved to LA, I loved the thought of being closer to him. After leaving behind my two sisters and parents in New York, it was nice to know that I had a family member nearby in California, even if it was a long drive. There are six years between Todd and me, and we've never spent more than a few weeks alone together. I lived with him and his wife, Diana, a few times while I was on tour with different Broadway shows. I loved it when I got to spend time with him and his boys— Oliver and Hudson. When I found out I was having a boy, I looked at them differently. Watched them play and interact, and studied their interests, trying to imagine what Elvis might be like when he was older. In some ways, I was the least close to Todd just because of our age difference and how little time we'd been able to spend together. But I knew he was the perfect person to come help. I couldn't wait to see him walk through the door.

Anna began making her plans, too.

"If you can come, please come," I had told her. "I really need my best friend here."

There were no flights that day; she had booked one for the next morning as soon as I had hung up with my parents. But there were no direct flights from Canton, Ohio. She had to connect in Atlanta and then fly to LA. It would be nine hours in the air, and she didn't even have a mask. At this time, you still couldn't buy toilet paper. There were no masks, no Lysol, no hand sanitizer. The stores were out of all dis-infectants, plastic gloves, goggles—even hazmat suits were completely sold out. There was nothing she could buy.

This was the height of COVID. Everyone was saying not to fly un-less it was an emergency; it was too dangerous to be around that many people. This was undoubtedly an emergency—but the only thing that could make this situation worse was someone else in the family get-ting the virus.

"What if I got it on the plane and then brought it to you and Elvis and Todd?" she said. "I would *never* forgive myself!"

There was nowhere she could quarantine for two weeks, and, to be honest, I needed her help—we didn't have two weeks.

She looked for help in the only place she could think of: Instagram. Anna and I already both had big social followings and we knew it was the easiest way to reach a lot of people quickly. She put up a story that said: "It is essential that I fly to Los Angeles as soon as possible. I am terrified to fly and have nothing to protect myself. If anyone can help me with a mask, gloves, goggles, anything, please DM me." She waited to see if anyone could spare a mask.

A friend from New York, Dante, called her five minutes later. I met Dante in musical theater school when I first moved to New York. He was also from Ohio, and we bonded instantly over being newbies to the city. He became my best friend that year, and we had stayed friends over the next decade in New York City, only growing closer as time went on. He has a heart of gold, the best smile in the world, and is just the kind of person you know you can count on.

"I have a full-face respirator. It's medical grade; I bought it months ago because I knew this was going to get bad. I'm sending it to you tomorrow."

Other offers came pouring in; people willing to give masks, gloves, painter coveralls, bleach wipes, everything imaginable. So Anna moved her flight to the end of the week and started driving around Ohio, picking up gloves, suits, and other gear from people willing to help. She assembled a makeshift hazmat suit a few days later and was ready to fly.

Rachel arrived an hour after Dr. William's call. She came in and instantly began doing whatever she could to help, which is her way. Rachel calls me "Posi" because one day I walked into rehearsal with a T-shirt that said THINK POSITIVE, wearing cupcake earrings to boot. She couldn't believe my choice of shirt for the grueling rehearsal day, and ever since she nicknamed me "Posi"—short for Positive. Rachel has taught me about gratitude for life and is a pillar of strength, serenity, and grace. She was the perfect person to have by my side as my world was crumbling down.

Now there were five of us in the house, and it was the weirdest feeling. No one wanted to be inside because we didn't know if we were even allowed to all be in the house. We were wondering how to handle the situation. That unease made everything worse. We didn't want to be in the house together because it felt unsafe, so Rachel stayed with me and Trevor and Zach left for a bit, eventually coming back but staying outside on the driveway.

Waiting for the phone to ring was terrifying. I knew that the next phone call would either be the news that Nick was on ECMO and stable for now, or that he hadn't survived and I had lost my husband. I couldn't sit still, or stop crying, or catch my breath. I went to Nick's closet and grabbed one of his oversized flannel shirts, anything to give me some comfort and make me feel as if he was with me.

Those hours passed so slowly—the longest three hours of my life, I think. I didn't want to go anywhere or do anything because I was waiting for the phone to ring. Rachel encouraged me to shower and clean up, so she straightened the house while I did that. Molly kept entertaining Elvis so I could be alone.

Finally, the phone rang. I picked it up, terrified of what the hospital would tell me.

Nick was on ECMO. The surgery had been a success.

He was going to be wheeled back to his room soon to rest. He was stable, for now. But we weren't in the clear yet. The doctor told me that every four hours now were important, testing whether Nick's body was accepting the machine.

I ran outside to tell the group that had gathered: Molly, Trevor, Zach, Zach's girlfriend, Florence, and Rachel's husband, Rickey. These friends would become my support group, a quarantine pod for the rest of the ride. We all cheered together, we cried, we were relieved. I grabbed Elvis and gave him the biggest hug and kiss. "Dada made it," I told him.

I called my parents, Lesley, and everyone else to let them know the good news.

I thanked God for saving Nick that day.

Up to this point, I had spoken only to the private health-care team, led by Dr. Ng. I didn't know I could call the hospital and talk to the nursing staff directly, or that there were other doctors treating Nick. But now I had the number for the nurses on the sixth floor. Private health still called each morning and evening with an update, but now I understood I could call the nurses and find out what was happening in real time.

All of a sudden, there were a lot more people involved in this production, and I had to think about it in a way that made sense to me . . .

I realized Dr. Ng was like the director, overseeing the whole show and making the big decisions. The ICU doctors, each brought in to share their expertise, were like the choreographer and conductor. And the nurses were like the cast; on their feet, performing eight shows a week.

By the end of the night, I was so emotionally exhausted from the day, I took a Xanax. It was such a relief to be able to sleep; I wasn't sure I'd be able to rest, and I really needed to. It was Good Friday; the symbolism of Nick's dying on Good Friday was not something I could overlook. It was such a strange coincidence: the first of many times his story aligned with biblical references. I went to bed with the phone in my hand, hoping I wouldn't hear from the hospital. But at two thirty in the morning, the phone rang.

The hospital needed my consent. Nick's kidneys were failing, and he needed to go on dialysis. I had heard of dialysis, I knew people who had been on it, but I really had no idea what it meant or what it does. I later learned it is very common when you are on a ventilator to be on dialysis, and even more common when you are also on ECMO. With machines running so much of your body, the organs just stop working and forget how to function on their own. It was the worst-case scenario. This meant more assistance, more machines, more recovery time, and more chance of complications. But there was no saying no—when you need dialysis, there isn't an alternative. I gave my consent and hung up the phone. I lay there in bed, praying, holding Elvis, and trying to get back to sleep. But the real-life nightmare kept me tossing and turning.

This day didn't feel real. Everything had changed so quickly, and I didn't understand how or why. Yesterday morning all was well, and he was about to come off the ventilator. Now he needed machines to support every major organ in order to keep him alive. I felt so helpless and terrified. I couldn't see him, visit him, or hold his hand. I thought about how I would think if it were me in there. It could have been. It could have been both of us. I eventually drifted off to sleep again but woke up several times throughout the night, worrying, wondering. I was holding on to the good things: he was stable, he was alive, and my brother was on his way. My friends had come to my rescue. I had Elvis.

The second I woke up, I called the hospital. I had to set up a password that would give me access to speak directly to his nurses to ensure it was me they were passing the confidential information to.

I went with "pizza," my brain always on bread.

The overnight nurse was still on duty when I called—the shift changed at seven every morning.

"Nick was stable through the night," she told me. "He is on a lot of medications, but his body is responding to the ECMO and the dialysis, so we're still looking at the four-hour periods of time to judge his progress."

I was relieved. It was the best I could hope for; he had made it through another four hours.

The flood of prayers that came my way overnight was incredible. People were posting on Instagram to please pray for Nick and sending love his way. New friends, old friends, neighbors, family. Prayer chains were going around and coming back to me. You don't always realize how many people you have in your life who really care about you until something happens, and suddenly everyone is so present, so giving and loving and willing to help. Nick was such a people person. He really loved his friends and family and always made a point to show people that. He would be the first person to offer support, listen to problems, RSVP to a wedding or birthday party, or be there to help you move apartments. He really cared about the people in his life, and they cared back. It was becoming more evident now than ever—and this was only the beginning. This outpouring of love was so uplifting to me; it made me feel as if I wasn't in this alone.

The phone rang again in the middle of the afternoon.

Now, and each day for the next three months, every time the phone rang, my world stopped. Whoever was with me knew to grab Elvis and take him outside so that it would be quiet in the house, and I would be able to hear every word clearly. As I answered the phone, I'd grab a pen and paper to write everything down, from a medical term or treatment I needed to look up, to what had happened in the last few hours so I could tell the group afterward.

"Everything was going well," they started. "However, one of the cannulas on the right side of Nick's body that connects to the ECMO machine is stopping the blood from flowing to Nick's right leg. So we have to take him into emergency surgery to try to fix it immediately. Do we have your consent?"

I almost dropped the phone as my body and brain went into shock again.

"*What?*" was all I could say.

My head was aching, and I started rambling off questions.

"Wait—what is a cannula? How is it affecting the blood flow? Is this common? Will it be okay? What is the surgery like?"

I was so confused. The tears started pouring out of me again, and I gave my consent because every minute was crucial at this point. When you're talking to the ICU, they deliver this information to you so calmly, so routinely, because it is routine for them. A typical day in the ICU is sudden surgeries, ups and downs, and big changes. But I didn't know this yet. I was new to all this, and receiving critical information like this—delivered so calmly and slowly—almost made it hard to believe it was happening. That was terrifying.

Luckily, as soon as I hung up the phone, Dr. Ng called me to explain further. Dr. Ng always had a way of making the situation seem normal, even okay. He explained what happened in a way I could understand.

"The ECMO machine is connected with four large cannulas, think of them as tubes. Two of them were inserted through Nick's groin. They are large and thick, arterial cannulas."

I would later learn the difference between venous and arterial, but at this point, I had no reference. The arterial is more dangerous because it can affect blood flow.

Dr. Ng continued, "It's important to get back in there right away and try to relieve the pressure that has built up so that we don't have a blood-flow issue to the bottom of Nick's right leg. So with your consent, we'll now go back into surgery to try to fix this. We'll call you as soon as it's over and Nick is back in his room."

Another consent, another surgery, another complication. It had been thirty-six hours. I looked for something to be thankful for: at least they were catching these complications quickly. They were taking care of them.

I hung up the phone a bit calmer, understanding the situation a little bit more. I started researching on Google. I wished instantly that I could unsee some of the things that came up: the images, the articles, the comments. It was horrifying. I learned what the cannulas are, what an ECMO machine looks like, what a blood-flow issue could possibly result in if not taken care of. It wasn't helping my anxiety, so I closed my computer and went outside to report to the group.

It was so hard to be at the center of this; I felt that right away. You have to live through the conversation with the doctor, which is awful and confusing. You're still trying to process it yourself, and then you have to go relay it, over and over again. First, I had to tell my Canyon support crew, then call Lesley, then call my parents, then update friends. You have to hear their reactions, which scares you even more, and field their questions, which you don't have the answers to. It's reliving everything over and over again. By the time I had finished updating everyone, there was usually another call and another round of updates due. It was mentally exhausting.

I became a zombie, emotionless while waiting for the phone to ring, but then tormented by the updates. From day one, the dichotomy between the hospital's version of events and Dr. Ng's became apparent. When the hospital called, the news sounded awful, grim, and cold. Then Dr. Ng called and, with his positive spin, made things seem okay. I was so up and down emotionally from that contrast that I never really knew

what to think, and that didn't change until the day I said goodbye to
Nick. It was such a hard reality of his case: different perspectives, different ideas, different outlooks, different versions of the same events. I
was continuously struggling with whom to believe, but I loved that Dr.
Ng lifted my spirits: "If we stay positive, we have options," and "This is
a marathon, not a sprint."

Finally, toward the end of the day, my brother arrived from San
Francisco. I didn't see him drive up the street, but I saw him walking toward me all of a sudden, and I ran right into his arms. I was so thankful
to see family. It is just a different feeling of security. All my friends met
Todd and seemed just as relieved as I was that he was here. They were
worried that I was living alone and glad that Todd would be staying
with me for a while.

"I have no plans to leave, Bigs," he said. It was music to my ears.

Everything felt happy for that second. Then the phone rang.

The world stopped.

I ran into the house.

"Good news, Amanda. The surgery went well. We were able to relieve
some of the pressure from the cannula, and he is looking okay for now."

Hallelujah! I fell to the floor and cried.

With the good news and Todd's arrival, the Canyon crew headed
back to their respective homes. Everyone needed to rest after what had
just happened. On her way out of the gate, Molly stopped to remind us
about the neighborhood concert later that night.

"Okay, so tonight, Jono is going to lead us in some music, and you
guys totally have to come. You can bring Elvis, and we'll be outside, and
it will be healing and so amazing," Molly said.

Todd had been to Laurel Canyon only once before; he had visited
Nick and me earlier that year when he met Elvis for the first time. He
enjoyed the community here, so I knew he would enjoy our Canyon music
nights.

The music nights were the first of several things Jono did for Laurel Canyon during this time to make our days brighter. He's what everyone dreams of for a neighbor. Jono has a massive garden and regularly delivered clay bowls full of fresh vegetables to people. Throughout the summer, he clipped bags of enormous, gorgeous squash blossoms to his fence next to a hand-painted FREE sign. He skateboards through the streets with his two little boys on either side of him and never has a bad word to say about anyone. His kindness truly radiates out and spreads to those around him.

At seven p.m., we put Elvis in his stroller and walked down to Jono's to sing, to "congregate" as well as possible while maintaining six feet of distance. We sang "Happy Birthday" to a sweet girl celebrating her COVID sweet sixteen and then "Lean on Me." We were all more than six feet apart from one another, but it still felt as if we were all holding hands. It was a gorgeous late-spring evening and the sun was setting; it almost felt as if we were transported back in time to 1965.

Singing with everyone that night was so uplifting for me. It was the first time I felt like I was really a part of my neighborhood, my community. I had never had that in New York City. People from afar were shouting to me, saying that they were praying for Nick, thinking of Elvis and me, and offering anything they could do to help. I felt fortunate to be there. My neighbors were all fantastic people, and Nick would have been so proud and happy to know that. The news had traveled fast through the Canyon, and they were ready to be there for one of their own.

Todd and I started to walk back up the hill heading home, and he was saying how lovely the singing had been, and how kind everyone was. He lives in Haight-Ashbury in San Francisco, also the "hippie" part of town, but with a very different vibe. Laurel Canyon is unlike anywhere else in the world, and I was happy Todd could sense that.

We looked down into the stroller at Elvis, who had his blanket up over his face. He quickly pulled it down and gave us both a huge smile.

"Oh my God, peek-a-boo!" I said. "Biggie, he's playing peek-a-boo for the first time! He's doing it on his own and showing off!"

I had been trying to teach Elvis to play peek-a-boo for weeks, but he just stared back at me blankly each time, clearly not getting it. Seeing him do it now for the first time, on his own, restored my heavy heart to feeling light. My face, which had been long and somber a moment earlier, was now wide with a grin.

Elvis had instantly changed the mood with one smile.

Todd and I said "peek-a-boo" repeatedly to him, and he kept playing along and giggling as we headed back to Brown Bear.

It was almost like he knew we really needed to laugh.

five

On Easter Sunday, I was praying for a resurrection.

I've never missed an Easter Sunday church service. No matter where I was, what city I was in, I made it to church on Easter. Growing up, we weren't allowed to skip church on Sunday for any reason—ever. My dad made sure we were all there each week, an entire pew full of the Kloots family, with neatly arranged hair and our best outfits on. Even as I got older, it didn't matter what event it was—my friend's thirteenth birthday party or the senior prom—if it fell on a Saturday night, I was not allowed to participate unless I promised I'd be at church bright and early the next morning with my family. During the last few months of living in New York, it was nice to return to that tradition. My sister Alison lived just a few blocks away, my parents across the hall, and Anna twenty blocks south. We'd all meet for church and take up a whole pew on a Sunday again, just like when I was a kid. Except now I was there with a kid of my own.

My brother and I did our own Easter service in the cabin with a small cross that he drew because we didn't have one there. We prayed and asked God to heal Nick. It was a day for miracles, and he needed one. We got on the phone with my parents and sisters in Ohio to update them. No one could even say Happy Easter to anyone else. It felt too weird to say happy *anything*. My parents asked me if I wanted them to come to LA. They felt like they should be there for me, and it was very difficult for them that they couldn't even hug me or do anything to help. But it was too risky for them. Todd was there—I had family. Anna's flight was in a week. I told them not to think about it. Just to pray for Nick.

My dad taught me to pray when I was little, and I've always followed his example. The first thing he does in the morning is make his coffee, grab something sweet, and settle into a chair with his Bible and a small Moleskine notebook. He writes as he prays, the first letter of every word he is saying. It helps him to focus on his prayers. I only learned about this recently, when his notebook was lying open on the table, and Anna saw it, picked it up, brought it to me with a stunned expression on her face, and said, "Amanda! Dad has his own secret code language!"

"Dad," we asked him, "you write in *code?*"

He explained it to us then, and we understood why every paragraph started with DJTYF:

"Dear Jesus, thank you for . . ."

Praying and asking people to pray with me were the only things I could do to help my husband at that point. I got on Instagram after our church service to ask everyone to continue praying for Nick, and to pray for two specific things: for him to wake up, and for the blood flow to normalize in his leg. Instagram stories had become the primary way I felt connected to everyone I couldn't be with.

Rachel had come over first thing in the morning to help us the way she always did: with a healing candle and palo santo. She and Todd immediately got to work reorganizing the house, getting rid of the copious number of boxes from deliveries, cleaning out the fridge, scrubbing down surfaces. Cleaning had been the last thing on my mind, and Brown Bear had become a bit of a disaster. It's an old cottage from the 1960s, so there's no dishwasher there, not a lot of counter space, and just a few small cabinets instead of a pantry. So there was always a pile of coffee cups and plates, deliveries of flowers and food all over the kitchen counters, and stacks of papers everywhere. It looked like a war zone, and having it organized was a nice breath of fresh air.

Suddenly, the house phone rang, and everyone stopped.

The nurse told me someone had called the Saperstein unit, asking if they could FaceTime with Nick. The nurse asked me if it was someone I knew and if I granted permission for that.

FaceTime with Nick? The idea had never occurred to me. I was so puzzled—I hadn't even known this was a possibility.

I said to her, "If *anyone* gets to FaceTime with Nick, it will be me! I would love to FaceTime with him!"

The nurse replied, "Oh, you haven't yet? Do you want to?"

I had felt so helpless for the last two weeks. I couldn't see him, talk to him, hold his hand. I couldn't enter the hospital; I couldn't meet his doctor. I couldn't pull a blanket up over him or push back his hair. I was his wife, the person who is supposed to care for him if anything happened—and I couldn't. I had replayed the last time I saw him in my head over and over again, wishing I had held his gaze longer. This sudden realization that I could FaceTime with him, that I could actually see my husband, caused me to instantly break down into a mess of tears.

"Yes!" I said.

I had to hang up, and she would call me back with an iPad the hospital used for FaceTiming with patients. I was anxious, and the seconds I waited felt like hours.

I knew that he was still sedated and that he wouldn't be able to respond. But I would be able to talk to him—he would hear me! Maybe my voice would wake him up. I fidgeted and paced as I waited for the nurse to call me back and connect us. I asked Rachel to be by my side for support. I was nervous, and she is a strong, calm energy. The phone rang, and I answered with video and found a nurse in full PPE on the other end. I was taken aback. I had not seen someone in the full gear yet—not even the person who came by to do my COVID test—and it was startling. It looked like a costume from a movie. She turned the camera to Nick and set it up so that she could do her work in the room while I talked to him.

A few times throughout this process, I was hit with the reality of what was going on and how severe it all was. Not being able to be in the hospital prevented the magnitude of the situation from fully sinking in. It let me stay in my own little world at Brown Bear, isolated with Elvis. This first day we FaceTimed, and I saw what he looked like in the hospital, it knocked the wind out of me. I was in shock seeing my husband—who normally weighs 225 pounds and always wears a contented smile—horizontal in a hospital bed, asleep. His face was visibly thinner, his hair was slicked back, his eyes were half open, and tubes hid much of his face.

I realized I had seen tubes like those before, but I couldn't place where. I remembered the tube in the nose connected to two round, white pads on either side of the face, which fed to a breathing machine. I racked my brain for why I knew that, and then it clicked. *Oh my God. Elvis.*

Elvis had been on a ventilator just a year before, in the NICU after his birth. I just didn't know it was a ventilator at the time. He had fluid in his lungs and couldn't breathe when he was born. Now Nick had fluid in his lungs and couldn't breathe. I could remember perfectly what Elvis looked like, all the little details of that machine that my baby boy had been hooked up to, and now my husband was on the adult-sized version. It was so similar it startled me.

I had thought the same thing in both moments: *my poor guy.*

It took fifty-six hours to bring Elvis into the world.

My contractions started June 8, my mother's seventy-second

birthday, in the early evening and got worse through the night. We woke up early the next morning and walked over to Mount Sinai Hospital because we lived only five blocks away. I was examined in triage and, much to my disappointment, sent home. I wasn't even one centimeter dilated after fifteen hours. I was told to go home, go on walks, eat food, take hot showers or baths, and breathe through the contractions. I could come back when they were three minutes apart, or if my water broke.

When you're nine months pregnant and contractions begin, you just want that baby out.

When you reach those final days, you want it to be over; you want to finally have your baby in your arms. I knew it would be only a few more hours, but I had already been waiting for forty weeks. I was done. I lay awake that whole night, tossing and turning, up and down, going to the bathroom, not being able to get comfortable, and feeling immense pain—as Nick lay beside me sleeping like a rock. At six in the morning, I tapped him on the shoulder in tears and said that I had to go in. I couldn't take the pain anymore.

These days, most women go into the hospital with a birth plan. "What's your birth plan?" asked every client I had seen throughout my pregnancy. Most women in New York have playlists, lighting requirements, meal plans, and a step-by-step guide typed out for how everything should go in their ideal world.

I didn't have any of that. I just wanted to have a safe birth and a healthy baby. I knew it was in God's hands; my birth plan was God's plan. I was just going to go with the flow. But I was beginning to question why His plan was taking so long. In retrospect, I'm glad I didn't have a plan, because it would not have gone the way I was hoping. Just like Nick's time in the ICU was full of twists and turns and complications, my labor was not easy or by the book.

They admitted me right to labor and delivery this time, but somehow, after thirty-two hours of labor, I was still only one centimeter dilated. I decided to do an epidural, and I was finally able to sleep. Four hours later, my water broke, and I was at four centimeters, but another three hours went by, and I only gained two centimeters, even with the Pitocin assisting the contractions. June 9 was the day of the Tony Awards. We couldn't get over the irony of our baby being born on Broadway's most important day! We put it on in the hospital room, and the doctor was sure that Elvis would be here by midnight. We were going to have a Tonys baby! But after three hours, the show was almost over, and I hadn't dilated one single centimeter more. The Tonys had wrapped, but our show was still in Act 1.

"Honey," I said to Nick, "I think the doctor is going to come back in here and suggest we do a C-section. I am okay with that. I am exhausted; it's been fifty hours now. I haven't eaten, and I am very uncomfortable. I need you to be okay with this."

Nick was devastated. He had the whole "Push, push, push" scene in his brain, and it took him a few minutes to rewrite the script. I found myself coaching him through our delivery instead of the other way around.

It took him a minute, but then he snapped back to reality. "Of course, baby," he said, "whatever we need to do to get Elvis here safely."

Sure enough, the doctor came in and suggested the C-section. We weren't in an emergency situation, but I wasn't dilating, and every time she pushed the Pitocin to a level eight, the baby's heart rate would drop. Pitocin goes to a level thirty, and we couldn't get past eight. Fifty-six hours had passed.

When you have a C-section, they place a drape midway down your body to maintain a sterile field, but there was a little window in the drape that they pulled down so I could see when Elvis came out. Nick was with me on the other side of the drape, anxiously awaiting the arrival of his son. When they were about to pull Elvis out, they positioned the window, and we saw our little boy for the first time.

Elvis Eduardo Cordero was born at 6:41 a.m., weighing seven pounds fifteen ounces. He was twenty inches long.

There's nothing like seeing your baby for the first time. It's overwhelming and so emotional to finally meet this little human you've been growing inside you.

When they pulled Elvis out, the umbilical cord was wrapped around his leg. This was why I wasn't dilating; the cord was preventing him from dropping down the birth canal. Thank God we didn't try to keep pushing; the cord could have cut off the blood supply to his leg. Elvis was taken to be cleaned, and we heard him cry for the first time. I'll never forget Nick said, "Baby, that cry will never sound as good as it does right now."

They brought Elvis over to me and laid him across my chest. "It's okay. It's okay. Hi, I love you. Honey, it's okay. Oh, I love you!" He was crying, so I just kept saying that over and over. "It's okay. I love you."

The nurse took Elvis from me to examine him and found something wasn't sounding right with his lungs. They said he had fluid in there, and they needed to take him to the NICU.

This is not what any new mother wants to hear, especially after fifty-six hours of labor.

"What?" I said, panicking. Then I rambled off questions.

"Is he okay? Is this serious?"

I was reassured that this was quite normal with C-section deliveries, that sometimes the baby has fluid in the lungs because of how they come out. During a vaginal birth, the fluid is squeezed out during the passage through the birth canal, but in a C-section, that doesn't happen. Hearing this was routine made me feel better, but I was also devastated. I just wanted to hold him.

I was wheeled to a recovery room; Nick stayed by my side as we waited for our room to be ready. I was utterly exhausted—both emotionally and physically. I felt like I'd been through a war. But I was charged with endorphins because I'd just given birth. Giving birth is the ultimate workout, and I had trained for it! I felt ready to do anything—but my recent surgery and stitches kept me weak and lying down. As soon as we arrived in our room, I asked the nurse when we could see our son, and she suggested that I take a rest and go in a few hours.

Hours? No way.

"Can I go right now?" I asked

Nick lifted me into the wheelchair, blood running down my leg, and he wheeled me to the NICU with the help of the nurse. This was the first time I was a patient in the hospital in my entire life—everything was very new to me. Before you can enter the NICU, you have to stop in a room outside to wash your hands. When we got through and saw Elvis, we couldn't believe our little guy. He had small pads on his face that connected tubes in his nose to a larger tube so that he could breathe. He had a tiny thing on his finger that was glowing blue and cotton wrapped around his head to keep everything in place. It was hard to see him through all that. He was just lying there in a little glass box, and all I wanted to do was grab him and cuddle him. Nick and I were crying with pride, but we were also scared.

Is he okay? I wondered. *What are all these machines?*

We reached through the small openings and grabbed his little fingers to hold his tiny hand. *Nice to meet you, Elvis.* For the next thirty-six hours, I did not leave his side except to shower, eat, and sleep. I wanted him to know I was right there. I knew he knew my scent, my voice.

It was the first time I fought a battle for the life of one of the men I loved. It would not be the last.

I quickly shook off the shock of seeing Nick for the first time. I had no other choice.

I knew he was there, even if his eyes weren't fully open, and I believed that he could hear me.

This was the first time Nick would hear my voice, the voice of anyone he knew, in days. He had no idea what had happened to him while he was sleeping, and if he could hear anything, he was probably terrified. He had now been off sedation for a couple of days, but he had not yet woken up.

I had to be strong for him, seem normal for him, and start talking.

Hi honey!

Nick, it's Amanda. I'm here, honey, right here. I love you, baby.

You look good, babes! You really do.

You're going to be okay. You have to wake up, though, Nick. We need you to open your eyes and wake up.

Honey, Todd came down from San Fran to be with Elvis and me. It's so nice to have him here, and Rachel is right here, too.

Baby, you got a whole lot of living to do, do you hear me?! A whole lot of living, but you gotta wake up.

I looked at Rachel.

I remembered that in a musical I sang a song that was called "Got A Lot O' Livin' To Do!" I couldn't remember where it was from, so I asked her to search it on Spotify. The first thing that came up was a song by Elvis Presley. Elvis! What were the chances of that?

We pressed play to listen, and it couldn't have been more perfect— the lyrics, the timing of finding it, and the fact that it was Elvis! We started singing the song at the top of our lungs to Nick through the phone. He always loved music, so it felt like a good thing to do for him. The hospital room was so quiet; he never sat in a calm room without music on. The nurse leaned into the camera and said, "His blood pressure is getting better! It's helping him, your singing!"

Music was helping Nick's blood pressure rise.

We sang with even more excitement as our voices got louder and louder. It felt so good to finally be able to do something to help him. I could see him now, play music for him, and sing. Hallelujah!

After I hung up the call, I had an idea. I didn't want to lose my adrenaline rush. I finally felt like I was able to do something good. I got on Instagram to rally my army. I explained what happened with Nick's blood pressure when I played him the song and asked everyone to join me later that day at three p.m. to all play, sing, and dance to Elvis Presley at the same time.

"Let's wake up Nick, everyone!" I said.

At three o'clock, we blasted it through the house—singing and dancing: Elvis, Todd, Rachel, Rickey, their daughter, and me. I was on a high, an energy boost that felt like I had just had ten Red Bulls and a shot of espresso. As soon as I posted a video of Elvis and me singing the song and thanking everyone for joining me, the flood of messages from people all over the world came in. So many people had joined me to sing and dance—even Priscilla Presley. She wrote to me that she was keeping Nick in her thoughts and prayers. I was speechless.

I lay in bed that night, thinking about what had happened, how hearing music helped Nick's blood pressure, how helping him had helped me. I knew we had to continue to sing every day. But if anything was going to wake him up, it would be the whole world singing one of *his* songs, not Elvis's. His dream was to be a rock star, to have people listen to his music.

We had had an argument not too long before when he was working on his music, and I'd said, "Honey, you're forty-one! How are you supposed to be a rock star now? The time has passed."

The world was upside down at the moment. All the rules were out the window. The possibilities seemed endless.

I knew my mission that night. I had to make Nick a rock star. He would wake up to find out that his dream had come true. I had to do three p.m. singing and dancing with the world again, but I had to play

"Live Your Life" next time. I wanted everyone to play one of Nick's original songs, and that one perfectly fit the bill. It was his first release, and the title couldn't have been more fitting.

I couldn't be at the hospital. I couldn't be by his side. I couldn't hold his hand.

But I could try to make him a rock star.

The next morning I announced it on Instagram and asked everyone to join me again at three p.m. I told them that we'd be singing one of Nick's original songs, "Live Your Life."

I was worried that no one would join in, especially with this unknown song.

But again at three o'clock, people all over the world joined me—dancing and singing along to a song they had never heard. People tagged me in the videos, so I saw babies, families, dogs, teenagers—everyone was singing, and it brought me so much joy. They were in the cars, in their house, in their yards, in bathtubs, on rooftops all over the world. It was stunning. I told people to start tagging their videos #wakeupnick, and the movement officially started.

I was alone. Nick was alone. But we were not alone. We had a little army cheering us on.

Everyone was quarantined at this point. Work gone, friends gone, lives completely changed. We all needed something to do, a part of our day when we "had" to do something. We also needed something to believe in, a hope that this all would pass. That something, for a lot of people, was #wakeupnick at three p.m. Something to look forward to—singing and dancing gave everyone something in their day, a story to follow—a community for them and me.

Todd, Elvis, and I drove to the outside of Cedars that day for the first time. It was Todd's idea; he suggested that we drive down to Cedars so that "you can do your thing," be as close to Nick as possible. My brother was the perfect companion to have that week. He stayed calm;

he was helpful—any idea to make the day better. By being outside the hospital, I felt one step closer. I stood outside the entrance and played "Live Your Life" as loud as I could, singing and dancing along. Going to the hospital became a part of my routine after that day. I didn't know exactly where his room was located, so I just kept my phone in the air and spun around.

The hospital reports were stable at the end of the day; nothing new had happened, and they say no news is good news in the ICU. But Dr. Ng was repeatedly telling me, "We've got to get him to wake up," and the concern in his voice grew a bit each time he said it. I begged for more prayers that evening from everyone following along. "I truly believe that if we all keep singing every day at three p.m., he'll hear us; he has to hear us! He'll wake up," I said.

Press requests started flying in, and I found myself a little over-whelmed. Nick was among the first of the young people in the United States to be admitted to the ICU with COVID, and I had spread the word. This was a story, and people wanted to share it. My managers and assistant quickly came to my aid and fielded all of the press requests for me since they knew that I didn't have the headspace at the time. The thought of adding another thing to my plate was impossible, but I decided to do a few interviews because I wanted to spread awareness about Nick; people needed to know his story.

Good Morning America was the first to do a beautiful segment on our story. I shared about three p.m., about "Live Your Life," and about my mission to wake him up.

That day, everyone was on board at three again! Most videos ended with people shouting, "Wake up, Nick, we're praying for you!"

I couldn't believe it when I watched them in bed that night. I couldn't fall asleep, so I looked through all the mentions and realized people were singing from all over the world: Miami, Argentina, Brazil, Baltimore, California, India, Germany, New York, Australia, Costa

Rica, Austria, Mexico City, Canada, Guatemala, Sweden, Dominican Republic, New Zealand, China, Texas, Georgia, London, Indonesia, Ohio, Venezuela, Jordan, Alabama, Bosnia, Denmark, and Moscow.

Every day, it seemed, more people were singing "Live Your Life."

Nick always considered himself an artist. He grew up doing theater, writing songs, playing instruments, and performing. He always knew he wanted to be onstage, and he was always the front man. At twenty years old, he left Ryerson University without graduating to start a band with his friends in Toronto; they were semi-successful. Nick and his friend Rohit wrote all the music and even sold some of their songs to Canadian television shows. But the new band wasn't lucrative enough to pay the bills, and gradually the band members left to pursue "real" jobs. Nick was a collaborator—he needed the energy and ideas of other like-minded people. So when the band broke up, he decided to get out of Toronto. He moved to New York City with his songbooks and $5,000 to give Broadway a try. He began auditioning and working at a record store for $8 an hour. Once he started getting roles on Broadway, they eclipsed everything else. But his own music was always on his mind—it just took a backseat.

When Nick and I started dating, he would play me songs over Skype until four a.m., and one of them was an early version of "Live Your Life." Nick would write many songs and never finish them: a verse here, a chorus there, half a line here, but never a full piece. "Live Your Life" was not complete; there were spots where no lyrics existed, and he would fill the space with ad-libs.

Years later, when we were married, we were in Hudson, New York, listening to his music. He played it again, still incomplete.

"That's it," I said, "we are finishing these lyrics tonight!"

We sat outside, opened a bottle of wine, and together wrote the rest of the lyrics. The song was finally finished. It still took him years to record it, mix it, and release it—but he did. He was so proud of himself, and after years of hearing this song, I was, too. His first single was out.

Pretty much from the start, Todd was saving my life daily. He had swooped in like Mary Poppins. I could barely manage the day-to-day responsibilities before he arrived, and with his help, everything was better. I didn't realize how much I needed help, how much I needed family until my brother was there. When I woke up, there would be a note on the coffee maker saying, "Coffee is ready for you," and the machine was loaded and ready to go; my hazelnut creamer was already out of the fridge and off to the side.

He accepted the multiple deliveries that did not stop coming; cooked me gourmet meals; watched Elvis whenever I needed time for a workout, a cry, or a nap. He made us homemade blueberry pancakes and warm muffins. One day I woke up to Todd making chicken stock for homemade chicken noodle soup. I could not believe his skills in the kitchen—I'd look in the fridge and see nothing, but he'd assemble a five-star meal with what he found inside.

He also took over sharing any updates with everyone so that after I spoke to the doctor or hospital, I wouldn't have to make five other calls filling in different family members and friends. I would have the phone on speaker, and he would record everything, transcribe the details into notes, and send out emails. It took so much of the burden off of me. He coordinated Elvis's Stroller Buddies so that we had a definite schedule each day, making it easy for me to plan times when I could do something for myself. With a teaspoon of sugar, he helped all the medicine to go down.

Sitting down to dinner each night after Elvis was in bed was something I looked forward to all day. We had lovely talks about life, marriage, jobs, and family. It was so nice to have this alone time with him, time we would never have had in ordinary life. It was a little blessing, a silver lining.

Meanwhile, the hospital reports were looking good. Nick's blood pressure was doing better. The dialysis was working; they were able to pull fluids out of his body, which helped with inflammation. His heart and lungs were getting stronger, which meant they'd be able to take him off ECMO in a day or two.

I felt invigorated. The world was singing and dancing, Nick was stable, and my brother was there. What a difference from the week before.

That afternoon, I came in to find my brother feeding Elvis homemade mashed sweet potatoes and talking to him like he was an adult.

"These, Elvito, are called sweet potatoes. They are like regular potatoes, only sweeter, and orange. They're special, and I think you're really going to like them."

Elvis spat out Todd's gourmet dinner instantly.

My heart flooded with love. It was so beautiful to see my brother bonding with Elvis, to provide Elvis with some male energy. Elvis loves his uncle Todd so much.

The hospital had called that day to tell me Nick was off the ECMO machine. His heart and lungs were doing well. Getting him off this machine was crucial; if you are on ECMO for too long, your body can forget how to work on its own. But the next few hours were critical. His heart and lungs had to work on their own for the first time in five days. He was off ECMO, but the blood clot in his right leg, caused by the cannula, was still an issue.

His leg was turning black, his calf was swelling, and they couldn't feel a heartbeat in his toe. They did a fasciotomy to release the pressure, which seemed to help, but getting blood to flow to his toes was still a daily concern.

Every day, usually two or three times a day, I would FaceTime with

Nick. Sometimes it was for only five minutes, other times it would be for an hour. It depended on the nurses on duty and what they had to do in the room. They were all so kind, so helpful, and so supportive of me.

I couldn't thank them enough for being with Nick and saving his life, but I told them how grateful I was over and over again when we talked.

My one request was that they keep music playing on the TV in his room. The type of music didn't matter—Nick loved all music! They agreed without issue.

It isn't easy FaceTiming with someone who can't respond. There were times I didn't know what to say, which made me feel so helpless and stupid. Then there were times that I couldn't stop chatting, telling him all sorts of things. Friends and new followers were giving me great suggestions on what to do to help wake him up. "He can hear you!" they said. "You have to speak loudly and command him to wake up. Tell him that he is in a fantasy world right now and that the things he sees aren't real life. Repeat over and over his full name, his address, his age, and who you are, your name."

So I did. I did all of this, every day, every time. I probably sounded crazy shouting into a computer screen:

YOUR NAME IS NICK CORDERO!

WAKE UP!

YOU HAVE TO WAKE UP!

I COMMAND YOU TO WAKE UP!

YOU ARE A FATHER!

YOU HAVE A SON, ELVIS!

YOU HAVE A WIFE, AMANDA!

YOU LIVE IN LOS ANGELES, IN LAUREL CANYON!

I tried really hard to stay strong on these FaceTime calls, but it was a challenge. If it was true that Nick could hear me, I didn't want him to hear me crying or sounding sad. I didn't want him to think we were scared or in danger. I wanted him to hear his strong wife telling him that she was okay, that Elvis was okay, and that he would be okay. So I started with that; then I would play music, a lot of the time his own music to jog his memory of who he was in case he had forgotten. I would tell him stories about Elvis and Todd and me and what we were doing every day. Elvis always provided a funny anecdote or two. I told him how people all over the world were singing his song every day at three p.m. "They're singing 'Live Your Life' for you to wake up, Nick! The whole world wants you to wake up! WAKE UP, NICK!"

To keep myself believing, I did everything I could. I prayed, I exercised, I wore socks with mantras on them to keep me positive. My arm slowly began to look like a game of Scrabble as it filled with handmade bead bracelets that spelled out ELVIS, NICK, LIVE YOUR LIFE, BREATHE, THANKFUL, LOVE, FAITH. I needed anything and everything to keep me smiling. After dinner, I would drift off to sleep. I never slept well, but I tried.

The next morning I woke up to news from Dr. Ng.

They had Nick on blood thinners to help the blood flow in his leg, but that had affected his blood pressure and caused internal bleeding. They had to take him off the blood thinners, but when they did that, the clotting was back in his right leg. It had become a battle to balance the prevention of clotting and the damage caused by the blood thinners, which got the blood flow down to his toes. His leg was dying, and his toes, foot, and calf were turning black.

"Unfortunately," he said, "we'll need to amputate Nick's leg."

It hit me like a ton of bricks. I couldn't even get the words out. My husband was going to lose his leg. He wasn't even awake to know what was going to happen. When he woke up, his leg would be gone.

I immediately thought of that moment. How he would react. He has been asleep through all of this, all these terrifying and scary things that have happened to him. He will wake up at some point and realize how much time has gone by. Realize all that he missed. Then he'll realize that he's missing one leg. I couldn't even imagine it.

He will be devastated, in shock.

I was devastated; I was in shock just thinking of it. A million thoughts went through my head: *He's an actor, a dancer. He relies on his body to work. What will he do? Will he still be able to work? Will he be in a wheelchair?*

"Is there no other way?" I asked Dr. Ng.

"To save his life, we need to remove his leg. We've tried everything."

That made the choice easy. It was his leg, or his life.

The surgeon would call me soon for my consent and walk me through the surgery, so I understood. They would try to save as much of his leg as possible, they assured me. They were hoping to cut the leg below his knee.

When I hung up the phone, I was crying. *My poor husband* was all I could think.

This had been a possibility, of course. I was aware that Nick's leg was decaying. I was aware this could be the outcome, but I wasn't prepared for it to be a reality. For what it meant for him, for us, for Elvis.

Would he be in a wheelchair? For how long?

Do I need to change our house renovations?

Can we even live in the house we bought?

What is life like with an amputee?

Until this day, I believed wholeheartedly that he would leave the hospital just as he had entered it. Now I knew he would not.

People who had survived COVID were posting their exits from the hospital on Instagram. It was called a "Code Rocky." All the doctors and nurses would line up and cheer as they left, mimicking a boxer's exit after winning a fight. I started watching them and was instantly in tears. I began fantasizing about Nick's grand exit. It was something good to cling to. He would get his Code Rocky.

He would leave the hospital, even if it was with only one leg.

We just needed the surgery to go smoothly. There was, of course, a chance of complications, just as there is with any surgery. Nick was already in a critical state, which made it more challenging.

We needed him to survive this surgery. We needed a miracle.

Coincidentally, "We Need a Miracle" is another song of Nick's. He had been working on it for months when we got to California and had just released it. So I played it loudly that day all through the house.

I could barely sleep that night and felt anxiety the minute I woke up. I didn't know what to do to make myself feel better, so I just kept blasting "We Need a Miracle" through the house. My brother, who was definitely sick of the song and was trying to work, never said a word or asked me to lower the volume. I asked for prayers from my army on Instagram.

"Please pray that I can see him. That I can hold his hand," I asked.

I knew this was impossible because of COVID restrictions, yet I still asked Dr. Ng every day, "Is there any way I can see Nick?" But I always got the same answer.

He never said no but reiterated how these are wild times, unexpected times, and that it wasn't up to him—and he would try his best to get me in.

It gave me some comfort even if I knew it was a shot in the dark. It wasn't a no. It was never a no from my positive doctor. I had become relentless in asking anyone I knew if I could somehow get in to the hospital. Those people asked people they knew to try to help me. A Broadway showgirl is not afraid of hearing "no," and never lets "no" deter her from trying again.

The phone rang that morning before Nick's surgery was scheduled. It was the hospital.

"Are you coming in?" the nurse asked.

"*What?*" I responded.

"This is Nick's nurse at Cedars-Sinai. I heard that you wanted to come in today?"

"Am I allowed to come in? Can I really come in?"

"It's hospital policy that before major surgery, you're allowed to visit the patient, and we also need you to sign consent forms. If you can be here at one o'clock, that would be good. He'll be getting prepped for surgery. You can stay for a short period of time, maybe thirty minutes. You'll have to wear full PPE. You can stand outside of Nick's room and look at him through a glass window. If that's okay with you, then yes, you can come to visit."

I couldn't even get the words out right. I was screaming, shouting, talking like I hadn't spoken English in years.

"I, of course! Oh my God. I will stand wherever you tell me to! I just want to see him! Thank you!"

I hung up the phone and screamed, "Todd! Todd! I get to go! I get to see him! They're letting me in!"

I was barely making sense, but he could tell what I meant and beamed.

"I'll drive you to the hospital, Mands."

Just at that moment, my sister Traci called to tell me it was Divine Mercy Sunday in the Catholic religion. I checked Instagram and had hundreds of the same message. People had seen my plea for a miracle, and my army had started writing in. I had never heard of Divine Mercy Sunday, so I quickly googled it. I grew up Lutheran, but we went to the Catholic church sometimes as kids because my mom grew up Catholic, and the Catholic church had services on Saturdays in case we couldn't make it on Sunday. I didn't identify with the Catholic religion, but I was on board when I heard this. Divine Mercy Sunday was the first Sunday after Easter and a day of miracles.

"The most miracles recorded are on this day," my sister said.

I am always looking for signs, and this was a sign.

What news to receive on this particular day. So I asked God for my miracle. We needed Nick to survive this surgery. We needed his Code Rocky!

"I know I'm not Catholic, Lord," I said, "but please!"

Todd and I grabbed Elvis, and we got in the car. Driving to Cedars-Sinai took seven minutes. There was no traffic; no one was out. We pulled up to the South Tower entrance, the same spot where I had sung and prayed every day for the last week.

"Tell them Nick Cordero, sixth floor, Saperstein," the nurse had said. The information desk would give me directions. I jumped out of the car, yelled goodbye to Todd, gave Elvis an enormous kiss, and ran into the hospital.

It had been twenty days since I'd seen Nick.

I was finally allowed in.

six

The instant I entered Nick's unit in the ICU I was struck by the stillness; for weeks now I had imagined it was going to look like a pivotal scene from an episode of *Grey's Anatomy*. Instead, the hallway was hushed, with just a few rooms that doctors moved in and out of routinely. This floor was for patients going to and from transplant surgeries. After Nick's last COVID test had come back negative, he had been moved off the COVID floor and brought here. He had a corner room with a smaller anteroom leading into it that was separated from the main part of the room by two large glass doors. This was an added safety precaution for the nurses, and a place where they could change in and out of PPE when treating him. They continued to wear it, and require the same from me, until his third and final test came back negative. The anteroom also had a desk and computer from which they could watch him twenty-four/seven.

The nurse led me to a window in the hallway where I saw into his room for the first time. This was day eighteen in the ICU, but the second I saw him, it felt like a reset to a new day one. Everything finally clicked, and I sensed the connection I had been missing, but at the same time, I felt like a fish out of water. I knew I was the only visitor on the floor that day—exposed as I stood there, crying my eyes out and silently praying. Nurses brought me boxes of tissues and asked me if

I wanted to sit down. But that was out of the question. If I sat, I could barely see Nick, and I knew he had no chance of seeing me.

The nurse on duty was named Theresa. She was older, experienced, and so kind and empathetic, the sort of nurse you want to be by your husband's side. She had FaceTimed with me previously, so I had "met" her before. By the end of the day, I'd started calling her "Mother Theresa" because of how she acted. She smiled at me when I told her her new nickname, and I thanked her for taking care of my husband. Theresa filled me in on how Nick was doing, what was happening, and what each machine in his room was doing. It helped so much to see things firsthand, but it also hurt. I knew nothing about anything at this point. That realization, seeing it all in front of my face, made me determined to learn. All I knew then was that my husband was about to lose his leg. His life was about to change forever. Our lives were about to change forever. He couldn't prepare himself for it, accept it, or choose it. I had to choose it for him.

I couldn't imagine not being the one to make such a life-altering call for myself. I knew he'd understand. When it's your leg or your life, you choose life. But I knew he'd be devastated. Nick used to be upset if he had a pimple! A by-product of being an actor is that you're forced to focus on your body, and how it moves and looks. This was going to be a big pill to swallow, and a huge adjustment for him. We didn't know any amputees. But looking at him, I was determined to find someone to talk to, someone whom Nick could talk to. He would need support.

After an hour of standing in the hallway, I think Theresa took pity on me.

"If you want to be closer," she said, "I can bring you into the area just outside Nick's room, but you'll have to get dressed in full PPE."

I was given a surgical gown to put over my sweat suit. I had two sets of gloves; one layer secured the gap between my gown and my wrist, and the other set went over the top for extra protection. I put a hairnet over my head, then my surgical mask, then a full-face shield on top of that. They took extreme precautions with my being in the hospital because they knew I was going home to Elvis. This whole process took at least five minutes, and I felt like an astronaut getting dressed to go into space. Now I look back and think how many doctors, nurses, and other health heroes were doing this every day, during twelve-hour-plus shifts, essentially spending all day in full PPE. It's unbelievable.

She led me inside, and I stared at Nick through the thick glass doors that separated us. It was the most horrible way to see someone you love. I wanted him to know that I was there, but since I wasn't allowed in, all I could do was scream when a nurse opened the door for a moment.

NICK! IT'S AMANDA!

I'M HERE, HONEY!

I LOVE YOU, HONEY!

WAKE UP, NICK! WAKE UP!

I shouted, hoping that he might hear me. After a time, in full PPE—with a robe, mask, and shield—I began feeling very light-headed. I hadn't eaten much that morning—there wasn't time to finish the eggs Todd had made me. It's not like a morsel of food would have stayed down anyway. After the nurse said I could come in, my stomach had instantly started churning.

Theresa asked me if I would like some time alone with Nick, which I so appreciated. Throughout the whole ninety-five days, it was strange to be in the hospital with your loved one while supervised all the time. It's such an intimate thing, such an emotional thing, to see your person like that. I would eventually grow used to the medical staff all around, but that first day it felt strange to talk to Nick and pray out loud and cry in front of nurses—despite how nice they were. So Theresa took a small break and left the room.

I finally pulled a chair up to the glass door and took a seat. I began praying, out loud, in a way that I never had before in my life. What was coming out of me felt like the Holy Spirit was with me, guiding my words.

"Put your angels around him, Lord. Give his body strength; help him to be okay. You are a miracle worker, and we need miracles. Help him to get through this, to eventually understand and accept this decision I had to make for him."

I cried through four masks, at least. They were soaked with snot. I was out of tissues. My eyes were bloodshot and puffy from the tears. The hospital had told me I would have only thirty minutes when I arrived, but it was going on two hours, and nobody was telling me to leave. I was so grateful for each extra minute. I tried to stay out of the way of anyone who entered the room, hoping they would forget I was there.

As surgery prep was amped up, nurses went in and out of his room more rapidly. The surgeon for the amputation was told I was there, so he came in to chat with me about the procedure. He explained that they would try to save as much of his leg as possible. They would try for a cut below his knee, and it should be a fairly routine surgery. But Nick was critically ill, and his body had been under a lot of stress and trauma already. There was a chance he might not survive. Having a doctor I didn't know tell me this after I'd spent two hours crying and praying, I went into shock. I hadn't fully connected the dots that Nick might not survive the surgery.

Through more tears, I signed the paperwork and gave Nick one last look before I left. I didn't know when or if I'd see him again. They told me this visit was a onetime exception.

My exit from Cedars was so different from my entrance. I had arrived full of adrenaline, running, searching, frantic. When I left, I was walking in slow motion, dizzy, foggy. Everything around me looked blurry, and if anyone tried to talk to me, I couldn't hear them. I was crying harder than when I'd been inside. My chest felt tight, and my body tense. I couldn't breathe properly; I couldn't stop crying. I was having a panic attack. My fingers fumbled for my phone as I desperately tried to dial Todd to tell him he could pick me up.

I was still sobbing, barely able to speak, when my brother arrived. As we drove home, I couldn't get the words out to tell him what I had just seen. Todd stayed so calm and collected. He drove us home and took Elvis right away so I could be alone. The surgery would hopefully not take more than three hours, and they would call me when it was over. I had strict instructions to undress immediately, put my clothes in the washing machine, and wash them at the hottest temperature. I had to take a hot shower and thoroughly scrub my entire body twice. This was to ensure that I didn't bring anything from the hospital into the house.

All week I had been on such a high. I was full of excitement and flooded with hope from all the dancing, singing, prayers, and press. *We are going to be okay*, I thought. There had not been a doubt in my mind that Nick would wake up, and walk out, and have his Code Rocky. That day, I finally crashed. Exhaustion overtook my mind, body, and soul, and I couldn't do anything but crawl into my bed, still wet from the shower, take a Xanax, and continue to cry until I fell asleep.

I had three hours to rest until I would get a call. I fell asleep praying that he would survive, that the only thing he would lose today was his leg.

Nick and I were in Grand Cayman on vacation the summer before our wedding. It was a much-needed week of rest and relaxation and time to connect while planning the wedding. We had agreed we wanted a small, intimate wedding with just our closest friends and family. We honestly couldn't afford anything bigger. So we spent the week writing out the ceremony, composing our vows, picking music, and working on the guest list. One evening I popped the question, "What should our first dance be? We have to do something fun! We're Broadway dancers!"

Nick wasn't sold on the idea. He *wasn't* a dancer and didn't want to do anything cheesy. His mind went to visions of YouTube videos and people trying to reenact famous scenes. But Nick rarely said no to me, and after a bottle of rosé, he had the idea of asking our Broadway friends Robyn and Clyde to choreograph a dance for us. I had toured with Robyn in *Spamalot* years prior, and Clyde had been in *Bullets over Broadway* with Nick and me. "I trust them," he said. I did, too. They were very talented and had a good sense of who Nick and I were as a couple.

A couple weeks before the wedding, we started our rehearsals. The song we chose, "It Had to Be You," Nick had sung in his audition for *Bullets over Broadway.* So it had special meaning to us, on top of having the perfect lyrics for a first-dance song. Robyn and Clyde had planned not a dance but more of an actual Broadway number—dramatic, thematic, and fun. We weren't just dancing, we were performing, and it was a blast. Nick and I realized in rehearsal that we had never danced together onstage, so this was going to be very special. Because of our respective heights, we were a perfect dancing pair, and—despite not being a dancer—Nick knew how to lead.

When we first got engaged, I had gone dress shopping right away. I didn't have a big budget for a dress, but I wanted to find something unique and special. I went to the Kleinfeld's sample sale and tried on the most unique dress I'd ever seen. It looked like a showgirl costume. It was a white romper, covered in details of lace, beads, and embroidery. Attached to the back was a long train that left the front exposed but back covered, so you could have a train and later take it off completely. It was a little wild, and I kind of loved that. No one I knew had ever worn a dress like that before. It was 70 percent off, and there was only one. At a sample sale, you have to take something precisely as it is. I couldn't leave it there; it was too unusual. So I bought it that day.

"My dress is not typical," I told Nick later. I felt as if I needed to warn him. Nick's visions of how big moments should look were usually rooted in tradition.

"It's a 'romper'? What's a romper?" he asked.

The mistake of buying your dress too early is that you keep seeing other dresses as you plan your wedding. A few weeks later, I still loved my dress, but thought maybe it was more of a reception look than a walking-down-the-aisle look. I had started to partner with a few brands on our wedding already, so I decided to reach out to some bridal gown shops in the city, too—just in case anyone was interested. I thought if I had someone reaching out on my behalf, it would look more official. But I didn't have a PR team or assistant yet to do that, so I wrote the emails from my sister Anna, who I pretended was my PR representative. "Fake it 'til you make it" has always been one of my mottos. A beautiful little boutique in the West Village wrote me back. They were interested in working with me and open to loaning a sample for just the ceremony and photos. I scheduled a meeting and asked Anna to come with me.

"Oh, by the way," I told Anna on the way to the shop, "I wrote this email and signed it as you, pretending you're my PR person coordinating all the media partners for the wedding. Ha! So if they say something about emailing, just go with it."

The boutique owner was an angel sent from God. She had the most stunning collection of dresses and offered to lend me whatever fit to walk down the aisle in. I tried on couture gown after couture gown, each one gorgeous. Each time I came out in one, I acted calm and normal in front of the girl so she would think I did this type of thing all the time—but then Anna and I would exchange glances in our secret language that said, *I can't believe this is happening! This is a total dream and makes no sense at all, but let's just go with it!*

I found my dress that day: a long-sleeved, backless, sheer dress made of shimmering gold tulle and covered in white, floral embroidery. It was classy but sexy. Classic, but modern. I would walk down the aisle in that and then change into my romper for our dance. It was fate—I could never have done our wedding dance in another outfit.

The night of our wedding, we had the dance floor cleared. To everyone's surprise, I did my "costume" change in true Broadway fashion. It was my Vera Ellen moment of the night. A nod to all the old movie musicals I loved watching as a little girl. Our dance was definitely a highlight of the night for us. The first dance always puts the couple in the spotlight—but this dance put us center stage on Broadway, with the crowd on their feet cheering. To our surprise, the next day it went viral. We were on all the Broadway websites and the *Daily Mail*, and we did national news interviews with *Inside Edition*. It was a moment in our lives I'll never forget.

As I started to wake up, I could hear Elvis and my brother in the front room playing.

"This, Elvito, is a ball. It's really neat because you can roll it, you can throw it, and one day you can kick it. But right now, you're probably just going to want to chew on it . . . Ah, yep. I was right."

I had been in such a deep sleep that even pushing the covers aside seemed to take all of my energy. I walked into the bathroom to look at my face. My eyes were so puffy they could barely open. The whites looked about half the size. Quarantine wasn't kind to any of us. We had grown-out roots, missed facials and tints. Staying inside had left us pale, and quarantine snacking had left us rounder. There was no need for makeup or styled hair. I felt as if I had never looked worse. I wasn't even sure who was staring back at me. Trauma transforms you, not just your inside but your outside, too. It's so hard to believe what is happening to you that it's hard to look in the mirror and confirm that you are, in fact, even *you*. You're no longer the *you* you know.

I went to Nick's side of the closet, wrapped myself in one of his oversized flannel shirts, and walked out to the front room. Elvis immediately lit up as he saw me, which filled my empty heart back to full.

His little smile has a way of healing pain. I scooped him up into a big hug and covered him in kisses. The hospital hadn't called yet. You don't know how to act when you're waiting for news like this, so Todd and I tried our best just to act normal. But inside, we were both on edge; every second felt like a lifetime. I tried to talk about other things, but my brain couldn't stop thinking, waiting for the phone to ring.

It was four hours after we got home when the hospital finally called. He was alive.

The surgery had gone as smoothly as possible. Nick didn't lose a lot of blood, which had been a concern, and the cut was clean and should heal nicely. But unfortunately, his leg was more damaged than they'd thought, so the cut was made above his knee instead of below his knee. I was upset to learn this; the night before I had researched both prosthetics and amputations, and I was familiar with the added challenge of not having a knee. But it didn't matter anymore. I was just relieved to know that the cut was clean, and that he was alive.

I hung up the phone with a massive sigh of relief. Todd let our family know, and I called Nick's mom. We were all thankful that everything was okay and that the surgery had gone well, with no complications. It wasn't a surgery anyone wanted to happen, but it was over and he was alive.

I shifted my brain to productivity mode now that I knew Nick was safe. There was no use sitting around being sad that he didn't have a leg. I had to start thinking about how I was going to help him through this, and I wanted to learn everything I could. By the time he woke up and could talk to me, I would have information and inspiring stories to share with him. A friend of mine had already put me in touch with an amputee who was willing to talk to me. I wanted to hear his story and pick his brain about what Nick might be feeling and thinking when he woke up. I also wanted to ask him about our new home. We were in the midst of renovations, and if Nick would be in a wheelchair going forward, I wanted to change things now. I needed help and advice. I wanted to get a head start on these changes so they would be in the works. That way, Nick wouldn't have to worry about them. I called the friend of a friend as soon as I could with my list of questions.

You learn so much in talking to people, hearing their stories.

He asked, "Did Nick have a below-the-knee or above-the-knee amputation?"

I said, "It ended up being above the knee. They were hoping that they could save his knee, but the leg was too damaged."

"Okay," he said, "he had an AK amputation, then."

I asked him to repeat himself because I didn't understand.

"If it's below the knee, it's called a BK, and if it's above the knee, it's called an AK."

AK. My initials.

AK. My fitness company

AK. My nickname, my logo, my identity.

It was too weird. Too much of a coincidence. It was almost . . . laughable. I knew when Nick woke up and I told him this story, he would say, "Of course. Of course I had an AK amputation."

I felt better the moment I hung up the phone. This man had a full life. It had required a change, an adjustment, and a learning curve, of course. But prosthetics are so advanced today that losing a limb would not stop Nick from doing anything that he wanted to do. I thought about Nick learning to tap: that moment I saw him exit the elevator on his way to classes, when I was wrapped in fur. He didn't think he could do it, yet his number in *Bullets over Broadway* "Taint Nobody's Business" stole the entire show. I thought about our wedding dance. How he had been hesitant to do it because "he wasn't a dancer," and how incredibly well it had turned out. He was a dancer, an amazing one, and he would dance again. *We* would dance again.

seven

Anna arrived late the next morning. Todd went to the airport to pick her up so that I could stay home with Elvis.

Nick was stable through the night. I, however, had been sleepless, yet again. I tried to sleep, but the nights terrified me. Enough bad news had come in the middle of the night that I always went to bed scared of what could happen while I slept. Most nights, I ended up sleeping with one eye open, my phone in my hand.

I had texted Anna as I was lying awake because I knew she was still up, packing.

"Sis, I apologize in advance. This is a very hard place to be right now. Very emotional. Very sad environment. However, if we get a miracle, then you'll be walking into a party! Bring the party!"

She replied. "I know, Mandy, and I'm ready. I'm coming to work and help and do whatever I can. I'm in battle mode. We're going to get through this. There's nothing I won't do for you."

I'm close to all my siblings in different ways. Anna is the youngest of the five of us. We were all born just a year or two apart, but then seven years later came Anna. So our seven-year age gap sounds extreme, but I am actually the closest sibling in age to her. There are fourteen years between Anna and Todd. Anna had moved to New York for college in

2007, and I lived there already with my ex-husband. Rather than spend time on campus trying to make friends, she had spent most of her free time with us. She came up for dinner all the time, making the trek from Chelsea, where her dorm was, to East Harlem, where we lived. She would end up staying the night on our couch because it was too late and too far to go home.

Over the last decade together in New York, Anna and I became not just sisters but best friends, and we always have fun together. We are always laughing, up to something silly, usually twinning by accident, and often seeking ways to indulge in something sweet. Being in Manhattan for the last decade and having unconventional jobs, we had spent more time together than I could have imagined. No matter what I did, Annie was there. At every show, every fitness class, and she was my plus-one on a series of little trips once I started traveling for work. She even taught my Rope Classes at Bandier for me in New York when I was out of town; I nicknamed her "little ak!"

We got to know each other inside out and upside down. We think alike and act alike and even sound so much alike that Anna could answer my phone and have a full conversation with Nick, and he wouldn't have a clue it wasn't me. During quarantine, we realized Anna could unlock my iPhone with her face. We had been through some hard times together, of course. Some minor health scares, my divorce, then her divorce. But nothing like this. Nothing that was this uncertain, this terrifying.

She flew to LA on April 20, wearing a full-face respirator, goggles from a child's science kit, latex gloves, and painters' coveralls over her clothing. She had only her carry-on bag, which was wrapped up in trash bags for protection, with holes poked through for the wheels. To make sure she did not risk touching anything on the fight, she took a sleeping pill when she boarded so that she would pass out and not need to eat, drink, or use the bathroom in transit. When she got out of the terminal, she disinfected her hands, stripped down to the leggings and T-shirt she wore underneath all the other layers, stashed everything in a bin, and sealed it shut. She put on a new N95, disinfected her hands again, got into the car next to Todd, exhausted, and said, "Biggie, hello!"

"Biggie" is how all of my siblings greet one another. Anna hadn't seen Todd in six months.

When she arrived at Brown Bear, I came to the screen door to say hello, but I couldn't hug her yet. I could just wave from the window. She left her bag outside until she could disinfect it and went around to the back entrance. In the house she undressed and went right into the hottest shower she could stand, scrubbing everything, while Todd grabbed the Lysol and began sanitizing everything she came with. This was the plan we had come up with on the advice of the doctors at the hospital to keep Todd, Elvis, and me safe.

She emerged with wet hair and a new surgical mask, and sporting one of my sweat suits.

I was wearing one of Nick's oversized denim shirts over my own sweat suit and had Elvis strapped to me.

It felt surreal to see her, and she felt the same looking at me. It had been only eight weeks since she was here last. We were all together in Malibu eating sushi without a care in the world.

It was three p.m. "You're just in time," I said. "Come sing 'Live Your Life' with me!"

"Oh, yay," she said, joining me, even though she didn't yet know all the words.

It was so nice to have my best friend back, to have someone to sing and dance alongside me.

When my Instagram Live was over, she surveyed the cabin . . .

"Is it okay if I organize a few things around here?" she asked.

We had been living in the guesthouse for the last seven months. It was very stylized when we arrived, with a lot of Zach's knickknacks and decor on shelves, surfaces, and walls. When you're a guest in someone's home, you never think of moving things around, so we worked around it. But we had accumulated a lot and also hadn't had time to organize. I had stacks of papers from the hospital on the credenza between an antique typewriter and a model motorcycle. The kitchen countertop real estate had been taken up by several appliances and gadgets, so Elvis's baby food jars and containers of Gerber Puffs, as well as all my supplies for morning coffee, were wedged wherever they could fit. Elvis's toys were scattered around the living room, and a sea of boxes that had been delivered—containing everything from bath salts to books to twelve varieties of artisanal honey—were stacked high in the entryway. Todd hadn't been able to get to them yet today, and a new mound had just arrived.

Anna was desperate to make herself useful. My whole family had been on the other side of the country, dying to get to me to help, and she was finally here. Anna is like me; she does not idle well. She needed to start something.

"Oh, sure, sister, do whatever you want," I said.

I went to lie down with Elvis, and she got to work. Todd, who finds immense joy in cleaning and organizing, was excited at the thought of this project.

"Ooh, cleaning! Count me in, Biggie!" he said.

"We're going to whip this place into shape." I heard them laugh as I walked down the hall.

"You start on the boxes and the pantry. I'll take care of the rest," Anna said.

When I emerged an hour later, they had completely changed everything.

Appliances were gone, and new ones were out I hadn't known existed. *We have a toaster oven?* I thought.

All the coffee stuff was moved and now in a neat little station. The pantry and cupboard for dishes had been swapped, reorganized, and cleaned out. All of the random knickknacks taking up surfaces were safely stored away under cabinets to create more space. The credenza was clear except for a stack of papers and an orchid; it was my new office. A "new item processing station" was established in the hallway for all the incoming things to be disinfected, sorted, then stored in the proper place. The laundry room was reorganized. Elvis's books and toys were sorted by type in neat little bins by the fireplace. The phone numbers for the hospital, which I had scribbled all over the back of a birthday card I frantically searched for each time I needed to call, had been written out neatly and taped to the wall by the phone. There was even a candle burning "New York City" scent. It looked like a whole new cabin.

From then on, I called Anna "Bibbidi-Bobbidi-Boo." She magically appeared here, and with a smile and a sparkle, made everything look shiny and new. She'd continue to Bibbidi-Bobbidi on a daily basis, never letting the house get messy for more than a few hours before she swooped in and waved her magic wand. She had also prepared lunch, anticipating I would be hungry when I got up from my nap.

The three of us established a rhythm that week that lasted for the next month. It was bizarre and beautiful and uniquely special. Three adult siblings, each with lives and families of their own, living together again with only the other two for company for the first time in twenty-five years. Todd's kids and wife were in San Francisco; Nick was in the hospital; and Anna was going through a divorce. We never fought; we never got angry at one another. We never put together a game plan or set up roles. We naturally just started taking care of one another and of Elvis. Todd and Anna were both able to put their jobs on hold, and mine was on hold, too. We had no priorities but keeping Elvis alive, fed, and happy, and doing the same for one another. We've always been so close that it didn't require a conversation to understand how to live like this and make it work. It came to us naturally.

There was already a lot of help in place at this point. Elvis had his

Stroller Buddies coming every day at eleven a.m. and five p.m. to take him for a walk. We could count on those hours of sanity. Matt Weaver was still doing daily grocery check-ins with us and would deliver whatever we needed. Rachel, Molly, Trevor, Zach, and Florence were all on standby for anything that might come up. The addition of Anna at Brown Bear rounded out this team perfectly, a final set of hands I knew I could rely on for anything, a mini-mom for Elvis for when I couldn't be there.

The next day, April 21, was a beautiful day, Nick was stable, and we were safely together. The report that morning was that everything was going well. They had lowered his blood pressure medication and vent assistance. His leg was healing nicely. The CT scans showed nothing new. It was cause for celebration.

When Elvis was on his eleven a.m. walk, Anna and I decided to do a workout in the driveway. This became a routine for us since when Elvis is around, there's no chance of getting a workout in. I had tried before—the result was a baby climbing on me and trying to breastfeed while I did crunches. Keeping healthy and on an endorphin high was essential to me. It's always more fun to work out with a buddy. We've been workout buddies for the last decade—whether we were taking Zumba at the New York Sports Club, or doing my classes at Bandier, or jumping rope out on the porch of our parents' home on Thanksgiving morning. It felt nice to be doing something familiar. Anna had always been front and center in my classes and knew all the moves.

Meanwhile, Todd was inside, making yet another breakfast and drinking coffee. It never ceased to amaze me how often and much my brother eats and still stays so slim. Anna and I would watch, green with envy and mildly annoyed, to be honest, as he prepared himself French toast just an hour after eating a croissant, eggs, and fruit. He's also a coffee snob, taking almost a full hour in the morning to grind, brew, and enjoy his morning cup. He would do it in front of Elvis, explaining all the steps to "teach him" how to make good coffee. I brew simple filter coffee at home, which I enjoy with a hefty pour of hazelnut creamer. It's ready in five minutes. I'm done with my one cup before Todd has finished grinding his fancy beans. Anna preferred Todd's coffee, but because his method took so long and she needed an immediate hit, she would start with a cup of my "gross coffee" and then would have another cup with Todd after our workout. I got into the habit of asking her before I started brewing, "You want my gross coffee today, or no?"

"Ugh," she'd sigh, glancing over at Todd, who had just begun to pour the beans into this tiny hand grinder. "Okay, I guess I'll have some of your gross."

The hour always passed too quickly, and before we knew it, Elvito was back.

"Oh no, not you," we said to him as he was wheeled back onto the driveway, "I thought we got rid of you," we'd tease. Then we smothered him in kisses as he laughed. Elvis was not sold on Auntie Anna yet, which crushed her. She had actually spent a lot of time with Elvis after he was born. But Todd had arrived the week before, and they had formed a quick bond in the chaos. He smiled and flirted with Anna that first week, but if she tried to take him from me or Todd, it was instant tears. Like with all babies, we all knew it would just take some time.

"Your pecking order is definitely Mom, then Uncle Todd, and I am a distant third choice," she said to Elvis. "But it's okay . . . I'll get there. I'll win you over, *petit* by *petit*, my Petit!"

Anna had been speaking French to Elvis since he was born, determined to teach him a few phrases while simultaneously practicing herself. She had nicknamed him Petit, the French word for "little," early on because he was so small and skinny. It was the perfect name for him.

Todd and I quickly adopted it, often reflecting on something naughty or cute he had done by saying, "Oh, that Petit . . ."

Nicknames run deep in our family, and once they are established,

they stick. We all call each other "Biggie," something Anna started calling Todd when she was a little girl; it stuck and grew to include all of
us. Todd was the original Biggie, but we all use it interchangeably now.

One of Nick's nicknames for Elvis was "Elvito Cordorito Monolito."

Nick's father's side is from Costa Rica, and he grew up going there
for vacations, so he knew a little Spanish. Adding "ito" to the end of a
word in Spanish is a way of making it cute; it, too, means "little."

So Nick's nickname for Elvis meant "my little Elvis, little Cordero,
my little life."

T he morning of Nick's thirty-fifth birthday we celebrated at the
Clinton St. Baking Company. The restaurant is famous in New
York for its pancakes and always has an enormous line, so we chatted as we waited. It was mid-September, and Nick was already talking
about going home to Canada for Canadian Thanksgiving. He was going
on and on about how excited he was to be going home and how he loved
being with his family. I had briefly met Lesley, Matt, and Amanda when
they visited him in New York—but I had never met his dad, Eduardo.
I had heard several little anecdotes, though: he came from Costa Rica,
and was a Latin man with a feisty personality and a lot of charisma.
Everyone in town knew him and loved him. He woke up each morning
and went to the grocery store and said hello to everyone who worked
there. In the house, he had his chair in the living room, which no one
else was allowed to sit in. He had a scarf he always wore when he sat
in it. With every meal, he ate rice and beans. Lesley and Eduardo met
while she was vacationing in Costa Rica. He was working at the hotel
she was staying in, and his first words to her upon arrival, after an ar-
duous trip, were, "Tired, baby?"

I remembered seeing how Nick interacted with his parents at the opening-night party of *Bullets over Broadway*. I could tell he loved and respected his parents, and I loved that about him.

Nick and I had been dating for only a few months. It was probably a little early to bring someone home for the holidays, but as he talked, I found myself dying for an invitation. I felt so close to him already and wanted to know more, and have a chance to get to know his family.

"I could go home with you . . . if you wanted," I finally said, getting up the courage to just invite myself.

Nick was caught off guard. You can't really say no to that.

I later learned that he hadn't brought someone home in a while. So when Lesley heard I was coming, she went to all kinds of trouble to make sure I would be comfortable. She redecorated the room downstairs where Nick and I would sleep; she asked Nick what "essentials" she should get for me at the grocery store; and she prepared several vegetarian meals for me ahead of time since Nick mistakenly told her that I didn't eat meat.

When we arrived, I got a tour of Hamilton, Nick's hometown. It's a quaint steel town that reminded me a lot of Canton, Ohio, where I grew up. Lesley and Eduardo took me past all the important landmarks in Nick's life: the school, the theater, the coffee shop. Even though these places were just buildings, seeing them gave me context for so many of Nick's stories. I was seeing a deeper layer of him, and I enjoyed every minute of it.

At their town house, we all cozied up in the front room in the evening to talk. I liked that they all were relaxed and just wanted to pass the time sitting, talking, and teasing one another. It's what my family would do. Eduardo was wearing his scarf and sitting in his chair, his spot. When I saw him in it, I had an inclination to go and sit next to him. He had a reputation for being tough, but I met him when he was older. He had softened up a bit—the way we all do.

Looking back, I was observing everything on this trip, learning about the Corderos. I wasn't a part of the family yet; I was taking them all in and I liked what I saw: Lesley and Eduardo's love for each other, their pride for their children. A true, loving bond between Nick and his siblings. A family that valued time together and leaned on one another. Honest conversation and advice.

But most important to me was that I could see how happy Nick was to be at home with his family.

I saw on that first trip to Hamilton all the ways that we were different, but also all the ways that we were similar. When my mom called to ask me how it was, I told her, "I think I could marry him."

I had told Anna to bring the party, and those first few days she was there were as close to a party as we got. Nick was stable and was improving a little without the stress his leg had been causing. They were continuing to reduce his blood pressure medicine and the support his ventilator was giving him daily. He was still not awake, and the concern as to why grew, but we were still in the early days. In our minds, it was never a question of *if*; it was *when*. In our minds, it was never a question of *would* he leave the hospital; it was *how*.

After twenty-one days in a coma, the doctors decided they wanted to do an MRI of his neck and spine. They would be able to see if there had been any damage to his brain that would explain why he hadn't woken up, or would show if he couldn't wake up. The MRI needed to come back clean. I was dreading this procedure because it would be either great news or terrible news. So I prayed, over and over again, that the results would be good, that there would be no critical damage to Nick's brain.

I continued to sing every day at three p.m., and every day I was so touched that more and more people worldwide joined me. It overwhelmed me that this was happening and that Nick didn't even know it.

I couldn't wait for him to wake up and realize it; it was his dream. Getting his music out there was the only way I could help him, and while it was unconventional help, it was beautiful. He would wake up and learn that he had missed weeks of his life and his son's life, that he had lost his leg, that it would be a long time before he could work again. But he would also learn that the whole world was singing "Live Your Life."

I continued to FaceTime with him every day to talk to him, sing to him, reassure him that we were all okay and he would be, too. I had been doing my FaceTimes with Nick while in the bedroom, away from everyone, because if I was near Elvis, he would cry or accidentally hang up the phone, trying to grab it.

It was beautiful—but hard and scary—to talk to him. It was also beautiful—but hard and scary—for Todd and Anna to listen to me.

I had a script I stuck to.

YOUR NAME IS NICK CORDERO!

NICK, THIS IS AMANDA, YOUR WIFE!

YOU HAVE A SON, ELVIS!

YOU HAVE TO WAKE UP, BABE!

OPEN THOSE PEEPERS!

WAKE UP, NICK. YOU CAN DO IT, HONEY!

Todd was used to it after a week, but the first time Anna heard it, she looked at Todd with tears in her eyes and said, "Biggie, this is heartbreaking." It's not easy to listen to someone you love in utter distress; not being able to do anything to relieve that distress, though, makes it even worse. It's like hearing your baby crying in the other room but knowing you can't go in there to save him.

When I was done, they always were there. I'd come back into the kitchen to find a meal, a clean place, a smiling baby, and my brother and sister. It didn't make it easy, but it helped me smile, too.

eight

When the hospital first let me in on the day of the surgery, I was told it would be a onetime exception. Los Angeles had been under a Safer at Home order since Friday, March 20, which stopped all nonessential activities outside of residences and prevented people from standard visits to the hospital. But after seeing others checking in at the visitors' desk alongside me that day, I realized that exceptions were being made each day to a small number of people. In normal times, anyone who wanted to come see a loved one would be allowed in during visiting hours. But now with the order, and safety precautions, visitors were only allowed in if they were on a list, and that list changed every day. So for the next two months I fought an ongoing battle with the administrative team at Cedars-Sinai to be on that list each day.

Security at the hospital was tight. Only one entrance was open, and you were not allowed to even pass through the doors if your name was not on the list of approved visitors. Then you had to have your temperature taken and put on a new surgical mask you were given at the door. You checked in at the desk, and were given a badge with the date.

Every morning when the nurse called with an update, I asked, "Would I be allowed to come in and visit my husband today, please?" I was friendly, kind, and hopeful.

It was always a gamble, and I was still counting on the answer being no.

They would answer, "Let me check; we'll call you back."

I didn't know who they were checking with, who was making the decisions in these early days.

I understood the hospital had procedures, and why they were in place. I respected and wanted to follow them. But Nick was COVID negative now; he was not on a COVID floor. I had seen how isolated and protected his room was, and how empty the hospital was. I was also COVID negative, and isolated at home with just Anna and Todd. Dr. Ng kept saying Nick needed to wake up, and I knew my presence in the room would help that happen. I had read several articles about how having a loved one present helps people wake up from a coma, and the nurses had noticed that when Nick was FaceTiming with me, his eyes were a little more open than usual.

I told them I would do whatever it took. I needed to be allowed in. I would take as much or as little time as they were willing to give.

The morning after his surgery, the answer was no. The next day, it was yes, and it stayed yes for a solid week, but I still had to call each morning to ask and then wait for the approval. It was the worst emotional roller coaster. On top of everything else going on, I had to beg and plead with the hospital each morning to put my name on the visitor list. It didn't make sense to me then how none of the outside factors were changing, but they had to think about it every day before they could render a decision.

But Dr. Ng said to me one day, "You know this is a whole new world; we're just kind of taking it day by day; debating and asking as we go, and figuring out what people are comfortable with."

Looking back, no one at that time knew what was right, what was safe, what to do. Each hospital had its own rules, and it was frustrating to learn that other people in other cities were able to visit their critical loved ones without question. But I understood that erring on the side of caution was the best option. They had to think about Nick's safety, my safety, the other patients on the floor, and the doctors, nurses, and hospital staff. Every time someone entered the hospital it presented a new threat. So the topic of visitors was up for debate each morning, and each morning I made my case. When a decision was made, I was called with the answer.

When the answer was yes, they would call me back and tell me what time to be there. It was always different, based on what was happening on the floor and with Nick that day. When I knew my visitation time, we planned the rest of our day around it. When the answer was no, I had to do my best to accept it since I couldn't change it. But I struggled to understand the reasoning. I always asked who was making the decisions, but everyone was pointing fingers in different directions, assigning the blame to a doctor, a nurse, someone in administration, or a board member. It made me angry because I was not requesting any exceptions or special treatment. I knew people were allowed to visit under certain circumstances. Nick was critical.

When permitted, visiting was a different story each time as the hospital tried to figure out this new protocol of how to keep everyone safe with limited protective gear available. Until Nick's final test came back negative, I had to get into full PPE, then I had to just wear a surgical mask. Sometimes they kicked me out after exactly an hour; sometimes I was allowed to stay all afternoon. I never knew in advance. So when I got permission to go, I'd sneak away so Elvis didn't see me leave, and Anna would take care of him while she cleaned, organized, and prepared dinner.

The only consistent thing was I didn't tell anyone I was there. It was difficult to keep this huge piece of information secret, but the hospital asked me to not publicize that I was visiting. I don't think that they were trying to hide their actions, but rather that given all the attention Nick and I had received, my sense was that they were worried about creating a media spectacle and frankly I was, too. I wanted to respect their wishes and maintain my own privacy where I could. While I was conflicted about keeping this information from an army of people cheering for us, I was also singularly focused on waking him up. And I knew that if there was anything that could do it, my presence could. I did not want to do anything to jeopardize my relationship with the hospital. They were putting their faith in me, and I was putting my faith in them, and we both felt it was best that I not publicize that I was there.

When I began sharing this story on Instagram, no one knew who Nick or I was. I was sharing his symptoms so that other people would know to look out for them, and asking people to sing and dance for my husband. I never imagined how critical he would become, how many people would end up following along, and all the things I would end up publicly sharing. So keeping some things private was important for me, for the doctors, and for Nick.

Even at the times I was most frustrated with the policies, I was all too aware of the privilege. I was lucky to get *any* time with Nick; so many families were cut off from loved ones completely. To think how many people had to spend their final moments alone is unimaginable. I was aware that each time I visited could be the last. So the first day I was allowed to visit again after the amputation, I came prepared to make sure Nick would never feel alone.

On Broadway, when you move into the theater, you immediately transform your dressing room into your second home. You bring a pillow, blanket, and family photos! You do anything you can to change the sterile space into your own. I wanted to make Nick's ICU room into a Broadway dressing room. I had asked Zach to print out photos from our last family shoot as big as he possibly could, so I could cover Nick's walls with posters. I told our family and friends to send more photos that I could add later. I brought a mini-speaker so I could play music.

When I got there, I was surprised to find out I could go all the way into his room. Nick had just had another negative COVID test, so they felt safe letting me in as long as I wore a gown and a mask. When they told me, I was shocked and thrilled. Looking at him through the glass had been so awful; I felt a million miles away. I was finally able to stand by his side. It was a huge relief—I finally felt like I could do something tangible.

It felt surreal to stand there and watch the machines keep my husband alive when, only three weeks before, he was standing next to me, perfectly healthy. They were trying to schedule a tracheostomy, a small incision where they create an artificial opening in your windpipe to enable you to breathe. That way they would be able to remove the mouth tube, which can cause tissue damage long term, and still be able to ventilate him mechanically. He'd still need a ventilator—Nick couldn't breathe on his own—but this setup would be more comfortable for him and get the ventilator tubes off his face. It would also make it easier to give him medications. But they couldn't do the surgery until he was more stable.

They were also trying to put in a feeding tube. Nick had already lost a significant amount of weight. It had been three weeks since he had eaten a regular meal, and you could see it in his face. As I stood next to him, I couldn't believe what just three weeks had done. He had swollen hands with black fingertips, a side effect of the blood pressure medication. What was visible of his face under the ventilator was sunken and drained of color. His right leg was now a bandaged stump, and the toes on his left leg were black like his fingertips. They told me he would probably lose a few of the tips, but it wouldn't prohibit him from using his foot.

It was so much to take in—all the things lost. But looking at him, I could tell that he was fighting inside. He wasn't giving up. I made peace with the things that had happened, and thanked God that he was alive and I was finally allowed to be with him.

It was, however, hard being alone in his room with no one to talk to. I didn't always know what to say to Nick, and you run out of ideas quickly when no one is responding. I wasn't sure if he knew I was there; he showed no signs of being aware. But I felt as if he could sense my presence. I kept telling him the same things over and over again. I assured him he was going to get his Code Rocky. I was committed to being positive and strong and to telling Nick that we were okay, even though, inside, I was far from it.

It was difficult to go when my time was up. I was leaving him there all alone, in a cold, quiet room. But I had a child to get home to—and when the hospital said it was time to go, it was time to go.

When Nick's dad's cancer spread, and the family knew he had only a few months to live, that changed everything for Nick. He was starring in *Waitress* on Broadway, and he and I actually weren't dating at the time. We had broken up that spring after deciding that our wants and needs were just too different.

Broadway's schedule is demanding and exhausting. You do seven shows per week with only Monday off, time you really need to rest your body and voice. But as soon as his dad fell ill, every other weekend Nick would fly back to Canada on Sunday evening after the matinee to spend Monday with his family, then fly back Tuesday morning to be there in time for a Tuesday-night show. He did this for weeks until his dad took a turn for the worse, and then he used his vacation time for the year to go home.

Though we weren't together, we kept in touch. Before he left he said to me, "I know we're not together, but I need all the friends I've got right now—and you're my best friend." So I checked on him and his family, and he kept me updated on how his dad was doing.

He spent the days in the hospital and didn't leave his dad's side, giving him sponge baths, feeding him meals, keeping him company, and having long talks. I could sense that this was changing him.

When he returned to New York after that trip home, he asked if he could take me on a date. I missed having him in my life, and I wanted to see him, so I agreed. In Manhattan, your date never picks you up—you just meet at your destination. But unbeknownst to me, Nick was now auditioning for the role of my husband, and he went all out.

He came down from his apartment in Washington Heights to pick me up and go right back uptown together to a jazz club on 108th and Broadway. We had drinks and dinner there while listening to live music. It was the kind of date that is both quintessentially New York City and quintessentially Nick. He opened doors and looked sharp, and he had a different air about him. At the end of the night, he walked me to the door of my building and said, "Amanda, I realize what's important now, and I've changed. I was being stubborn, and I have an ego, and I can't lose you. I told my dad that I want to marry you, and he said to me, 'You marry that woman.'"

I stood there stunned. It's what every girl wants to hear.

"Oh, okay . . ." I eventually replied, wanting to believe him but knowing it's a lot easier for someone to say he's changed than actually to do it.

"Amanda, I'm going to fight for you," he said, and with that bold declaration, he kissed me good night and went home.

We went on a few more official dates like this, during which I pretended that he had to "win me back"—but really, from the second he finished that monologue, I was done for. We were fully back together a few weeks later, getting ice cream down in the East Village, when his mom called to tell him his dad had passed away. We flew to Canada together the next morning.

Eduardo had a beautiful memorial to celebrate his life, and it was there that I saw how different Nick really was. He was the man of the house now, and he stepped into the role despite how difficult it was. I was in awe of him as he took care of his mom, his brother, and his sister that weekend. He gave a beautiful speech to honor his dad's memory, celebrating his dad's life instead of mourning his loss, and stayed strong. I was equally in awe of Lesley, who threw a huge party at the house after the service. She hosted, and cooked, and made sure everyone was fed and comfortable. She had just lost the love of her life, and yet there she was, taking care of others and smiling. I was so glad I was there beside them, and I remember thinking, *What a family of fighters.*

Nick truly had changed. He was able to look at life and at himself and realize not only that he needed to change, but, more important, he wanted to change.

The older we get, the more stubborn we become—and change is a hard thing. His desire to evolve, to fight for his family, and to fight for me filled me with so much respect for him and made me fall even deeper in love with him.

When I got back to the house, it was always sparkling clean. The morning mess had been cleared. Elvis was fed, happy, and in clean clothes. Dinner plans were in motion, and a candle was burning. I had to sneak in through the back door, hop right into the shower, and then emerge switched into mom mode. It was the oddest mindset reversal. I'd leave the hospital sad, exhausted, and defeated, and on the way home I had to shift into strong, happy, and playful for Elvis. I was never allowed to stay at the hospital very long, so I was back in time to feed him dinner and put him to bed. I had established a routine with him, and as long as I did each step, he went right down without a fuss.

First, he got a bath in the sink as quickly as possible because he hated them. Anna usually helped me because it's far easier to control a slippery ten-month-old when you are two instead of one. Then I wrapped him in a towel and took him to the changing table to get lotion and a nighttime diaper. While I did that, Anna picked out his PJs from the other room. He looked cute in everything, but we had our favorites: Matching lemon-print ones my friend had sent us, light blue long johns that had a mini-mock-turtleneck top, and a footed onesie with cookies and glasses of milk all over it. While I put on his jammies, she combed his wet hair with a little silver brush from Tiffany that Dante had given me for my baby shower. Then I'd sit in the rocking chair, and Anna would turn off all the lights and close the door. I rocked him while I breastfed, sang him "La La Lu," and put him in his crib.

There was always dinner waiting for me when I walked into the kitchen. With Elvis now asleep, I could enjoy a few sips of wine in the evening knowing that I did not have to breastfeed again for several hours. As much as I wanted to have a few glasses, I always had to think of him first.

The next morning I FaceTimed Nick over breakfast, so I stayed in the kitchen rather than retreating to my bedroom. I was still in my lemon-print PJs, slippers, and crazy hair from sleeping. No one but me had really seen what he looked like on the other side of the screen yet. I had described it, but it's different in person, and it was quite a shock.

My siblings didn't miss a beat. Anna sat down next to me, smiling at the screen, and said, "Brother! So nice to see you! We really miss you around here! You've got to wake up and come back. It's not as fun without you!"

After my script, I was out of words to say, so I started playing more music, and on the theme of Code Rocky, I decided to go with "Eye of the Tiger."

I sang it to him, at the top of my lungs, though I didn't know all the words.

"Bamp, bamp bamp bamp," I sang along with the famous opening.

He was moving his eyes a bit, almost as if he was trying to acknowledge all the positive affirmations.

"Come on, Nick, you can do it, honey. Wake up, sweetheart. Open those eyes, honey. I love you. I love you, Nick—you can do it!"

These calls were like training sessions. I felt like I was back at the studio trying to motivate someone through a workout they thought was impossible. Like a private session, the phone calls took a lot out of me, too. But I never quit, and when my "private" was over, I had to move on to my next client: Elvis.

I'd go from FaceTiming with Nick to crawling around on the floor with Elvis. I wanted to spend as much time with him in the morning as possible, since I never knew where the rest of the day would take me. I could end up in the hospital for hours, or I could end up home all day.

As I waited to learn the results of Nick's MRI, I found hope in unexpected places. Ever since I'd gone public with Nick's story, I'd gotten many messages on Instagram from people asking me if I wanted to speak to their healer, do a guided meditation, have a Reiki session, or talk to a medium. Everyone offered what they could. Even though I didn't necessarily believe in any of those things, I was intrigued. I was desperate to try anything that might help, and I didn't think people sending healing energy to Nick would be a bad idea. My Christian faith made me a tad hesitant, but I decided to talk to a few people. While all the healers, therapists, and other people who had offered help were well intentioned, I had spoken to them only once. I had strange feelings about them, or guilty feelings, or just didn't find their methods helpful—all but one woman.

I was introduced to Steph through my client Chandra. When I moved to LA, Chandra started training with me, and I instantly adored her. She drove an hour each way to do a private session with me and was the kindest client I had met on the West Coast. When Nick was first admitted to the hospital, she had been the first to send me meals, a neck massager, and other things she thought could be of help. Chandra offered to babysit Elvis, to help me clean—anything I needed. She told me one day that she had shared my story with her cousin who lived in Hawaii. When her cousin heard Nick's story, she felt an instant, inexplicable connection to him.

"I'm sure this might sound crazy," Chandra warned, "but if you want to talk to her, I can give you her number. If you don't, that is totally fine! But either way, she's praying for you both and just wants to help."

At this point, I wanted to talk to anyone and everyone who might have information on Nick. I decided to call her and learn more about her. I at least wanted to hear her out and see what she had to say.

She lives in Hawaii on the island of Molokai, which is known in folklore to have magical, healing powers. She is a mom and wife and was the first to debunk her own claims. She said she couldn't explain it, but this had happened to her once before. She would suddenly feel the need to pray for someone, and when she did, she would be able to sense or see what that person needed. "I don't do this, I don't advertise it or even share it, but I had to share it with you. I know you can't talk to him, and this virus has so many unknowns. If you want, I can tell you what I feel, what I sense when it comes over me. Only if you want," she said.

We started texting, and in the beginning, I assigned very little weight to her messages. But she kept talking about seeing dark areas that needed to be cleared, and asking me where Nick needed help. I learned that in energy healing, the healer believes they can channel positive energy into a patient where it is needed most to effect results. The only thing I could tell her was that we were waiting for an MRI to give us a greater understanding of Nick's brain. He hadn't woken up yet, and they had found two mini-strokes from the CT scans. The MRI would tell us exactly where they were and the extent of the damage they had caused.

She told me she was being led to a part of Nick's brain near the back of his head.

"I'm not a doctor," she wrote. "I don't know what this is, but I see dark matter here that needs to be cleared." She sent a picture of the brain and circled a tiny area at the bottom of the head near the top of the neck.

Scheduling Nick's MRI had been dependent on getting him off blood pressure medication. When it finally happened that week, I heard from Dr. Ng a few hours later. We had a new system when the phone rang now. Todd pulled out a notepad to jot things down and write questions that came to mind to ask the doctor. Anna hit record on her phone, starting a voice memo to record the entire conversation. I answered, put the doctor on speakerphone, and waited for the news.

The MRI had shown in more detail the two mini-strokes in Nick's brain, which had likely occurred when he "died" for two minutes. It's common for this to happen because when your heart stops, oxygen stops flowing to your brain. One was tiny, there was not a lot of damage that they could see, and it was nothing to be concerned about, in their opinion. The other was a bit larger, and he was uncertain what the effects would be.

"There's a chance this is why he hasn't woken up yet," he said. "But we don't think it's why, and there's no reason to believe that he won't wake up! There was no catastrophic damage visible, which is the best news possible. So we believe he will wake up—it's just going to take time," Dr. Ng said. "It might take him a month? Definitely a while. This is much more of a marathon than a sprint. We just have to wait."

This reassured me, of course; his MRI had come back basically as good as it could be. But it was also a small setback; it gave us no answers as to when he would wake up, or why he hadn't yet. Our only answer was we had to wait.

Another *month*, I thought. Dr. Ng had spent the last week telling me the importance of his waking up. Every day he spent on a vent was dangerous, so what would happen to his body after another month?

Dr. Ng had said the strokes were in a part of the brain called the pons.

"Sorry, how do you spell that?" I asked. I wanted to research it the minute we hung up. "The paws?"

"P-o-n-s," he said.

The pons, I learned, is the bottom stem of the brain that controls speech, chewing, and a few other vital functions. They wouldn't know the extent to which Nick was affected until he woke up, but they could tell by the size of the strokes that rehab could probably address any issues.

I hung up the phone and yelled, "Hallelujah!" At the same time, Todd and Anna yelled, "Yes!"

There was no critical brain damage. There was no reason he would not wake up.

We hugged each other tight and cried, and then they started to spread the news.

Anna had set up a WhatsApp group with our immediate family, Nick's family, and our closest friends—we called it Code Rocky—and she offered to take over all the updates and put them in one place so I wasn't burdened with it. She recorded every call we got from the doctors and sent them to the group as soon as it was over. Now everyone could hear the update from Dr. Ng in his own words. While she did that, Todd went to grab Elvis, who was returning from his walk, and I sat down and googled, "Where is the pons?" A diagram of the brain came up, showing the pons in the bottom, near the neck. My mind instantly flashed back to a few days before—the picture Steph had sent me of the brain, with an area circled where she had felt Nick needed healing. It was the pons.

I had chills. I told Anna and Todd, who were just as skeptical as I was of anyone who claimed they could talk to, or "see," Nick. It could have been a coincidence, but it was certainly a weird one. Steph said she would continue to pray and tell me whatever she felt, and now I was a little more invested in her visions than before. I always believed it was God, and only God, who had the power to heal Nick, and I never felt as if Steph was a threat to my faith. She always said that she achieved these visions through prayer, and that God led her to see and pray for him. Her ways were rooted in the faith, so I wasn't afraid.

"God and God alone has the power to heal him, Amanda," she said one day. "He wants Nick to know that."

That night, I got a call from the pastor of the Bel Air Church. I had never attended, but my friend had given her my number with my consent. She called me to let me know the church was praying for me and asked if she could pray for me over the phone. I hadn't found a church in LA yet, so it felt wonderful to have this connection, to know an entire congregation was praying for Nick and me, as if we were members of the church family.

She asked me if I knew that Cordero meant "lamb," and I said that I did. We had made it the theme of Elvis's nursery; he was our little Cordero, our little lamb.

"Amanda," she asked, "do you know the parable of the Good Shepherd?"

I had grown up going to Sunday school and knew all the stories, but I couldn't recall the exact details, so I asked her to remind me.

It's the story of a shepherd tending to his sheep, and one goes missing. Rather than letting him be lost, he goes after him, determined to save him. When he finds him, far from the herd, he carries him back to the rest of the flock on his own shoulders.

It's talked about again in the Gospel of Luke. Jesus asks a crowd:

Which of you men, if you had one hundred sheep and lost one of them, wouldn't leave the ninety-nine in the wilderness and go after the one that was lost until he found it? When he has found it, he carries it on his shoulders, rejoicing. When he comes home, he calls together his friends and his neighbors, saying to them, "Rejoice with me, for I have

found my sheep which was lost!" I tell you that even so there will be
more joy in heaven over one sinner who repents than over ninety-nine
righteous people who need no repentance.

"It's a parable about trusting in God as our Savior and knowing
that he will come to find you if you are lost and carry you home himself," she said.

I was in tears by the time she finished.

Nick did not believe in God. It was something we struggled with.
He believed in a greater power, in something, but he was not a Christian. When I googled this quickly, the first thing that came up was an
image of a shepherd, carrying a lamb on his shoulders—a lamb with a
wounded leg.

I got on Instagram, overwhelmed and in disbelief at the parallels.
First, Nick had "died" on Good Friday. He made it through Easter
weekend and stabilized on Easter Sunday. On Divine Mercy Sunday,
I prayed for a miracle, and Nick survived the surgery that could have
killed him. Now this parable. It shook me to my core.

I couldn't help but feel that God was trying to talk to him. I got on
Instagram right away and told this story. Moments after I had finished,
Nick's mom, Lesley, called me.

"Amanda," she said, "I just saw your story. In the corner of my living room, where I'm sitting right now, is a statue that Eduardo and I
bought a few years ago. We were weirdly drawn to it."

She is not a Christian, but she is an artist and art lover.

"What is it, Mom?" I asked.

"It's a statue of a man carrying a lamb on his shoulders. It's called
The Good Shepherd."

nine

With three of us in the house now, everything was more manageable. Someone could be on Elvis duty; someone could be cooking, cleaning, and organizing; and someone could be working, resting, or exercising. Anna and Todd seemed to know what I needed even before I did. I'd come out of the bedroom thinking about grabbing a snack, only to find Anna making me avocado toast. I'd remind myself I needed to call the contractor, then hear Todd on the phone with him, coordinating everything. I'd remember I was out of creamer, only to realize they'd already picked up another bottle on a grocery run to the Canyon Country Store because they knew I was low.

Things felt calmer, and throughout the day, we found ways to laugh. It's who we are deep down—positive people who love each other dearly and understand that laughter is the best medicine. So we laughed about the mountains of boxes that accumulated. We laughed about how every call you make in Laurel Canyon drops and leaves you on the line yelling, "Can you hear me, hello? Are you there? Hello? Shoot!" We laughed about how we had started to dread deliveries of bouquets because Brown Bear had begun to look more like a flower shop than a home, and we had run out of surfaces for all of the vases. We laughed about Elvis constantly trying to break into the liquor cabinet.

Elvis brought the most stress *and* the most laughter to our day. You can't take your eyes off a ten-month-old for even a minute. Todd had two boys of his own, but they were now ten and eight; it had been years since he had taken care of a baby. I was a new mom. I was still learning everything and going through it for the first time. Anna had never had a baby; her only experience was our other nieces and nephews. We laughed about this strange reality so much that the first week as we adjusted to it: three adults with different lives, together in the same house, trying to take care of a baby.

One morning as Todd held a spoonful of baby food in front of Elvis's face and said, "Try it, Edward, you'll like it." It was a quote from a movie we'd loved as kids.

"Oh my gosh," Anna realized, "we are *living Three Men and a Baby.*"

My parents raised us to be one another's best friends. We spent a lot of time together as a family and were rarely allowed to have friends over or do sleepovers as kids; there were already five children in the house. We grew up playing together, taking baton classes together, and doing everything with one another. When Anna was born in 1989, she became our live baby doll and cemented our time together as siblings even more. When we got home from school, we all rushed inside to play with Anna. It was so exciting to have a baby sister that we fought over who got to hold her first and for how long. We dressed her up, and we played with her all evening, all of us together, instead of going our separate ways.

This didn't waver through the years, even as we got older. We spent our time together. We took family vacations, ate dinner every night at our round kitchen table, and went on surprise, family-fun days my dad called Uncle Wiggily Adventures. We had many traditions, like family movie nights.

It was rare that all five of us agreed on something, so the odds of agreeing on the same movie to rent at Video Safari were slim. To avoid arguments, my dad created a rotation: each week, one kid got to go with my parents and choose the film, and everyone else had to "like it, or lump it," in his words.

Usually, no matter who chose the film, the selection was a Disney movie from the "Family" section, like *Mary Poppins* or *The Sound of Music*, and there might be some initial grunts upon the reveal. Still, everyone was usually more or less okay with it. The one exception was when my oldest sister, Traci, was up for her turn. Everyone dreaded it because she always chose *Black Beauty*!

We had a few family staples: *The Sandlot, A League of Their Own, The Princess Bride*. But our favorite was *Three Men and a Baby*.

Released in 1987, *Three Men and a Baby* follows three bachelors—Michael, Peter, and Jack—whose lives spiral into chaos as they suddenly have to take care of a baby named Mary. She's Jack's child and is left on their doorstep with no explanation, and they have to try to take care of her while juggling their personal lives and also getting caught up in a drug hustle. Their naivety and unconventional child-care methods are hilarious, and the movie was so popular there was a sequel years later called *Three Men and a Little Lady*. Everyone in my family can recite every word to both films. We grew up on them and quote them all the time still.

We were just like the movie—but as siblings instead of bachelors. *Three Sibs and a Baby*.

With nothing to do that evening after dinner, we decided to watch both movies. In the second film, Michael, Peter, and Jack do a bedtime "rap" for Mary, which we instantly decided we needed to adapt and perform for Elvis.

We were in hysterics throughout the whole process. Todd has always been clever with words; Anna is a writer; and I'm a performer! The words came together perfectly, and I looked for costumes in Nick's closet to match the outfits the guys wore in the film. Everything meshed seamlessly. We rehearsed the song and choreography the whole night so we'd be ready to film it the next day and show it to Nick.

We filmed "Elvis Wanted a Rap Song" and then took it a step further by re-creating the movie poster in Photoshop. Our lyrics were . . . original . . . to say the least.

Amanda
Introducing Amanda, Anna, and Biggie
Your rhymin' 3 sibs rapping the Elvis diddy.
Just a little baby, you need your sleep.
Don't wanna hear no cries whining about somethin' to eat.
Break it down . . .
Light's out.

Anna
I was living in Paris; they were husbands and wives.
Then the coronavirus came and changed our lives.

Todd
We're dedicated siblings, besties, and friends,
Together in LA, until this thing ends.
Say, Elvis, did you get your bath?

Anna
Say, Elvis, did you have a boob?

Amanda
Now Anna start cooking, Todd cue a flick,

Anna
Mands start dancing to #WakeUpNick!

ALL
To little baby Elvis we say please,
Just close your eyes and cop some Zs . . .

This was the first pure, silly fun I had had in weeks. It felt so good to laugh that hard. I had already done my fair share of goofy things to entertain Elvis, but this took it up a notch. We sent it to our whole family; it brought some much-needed laughter to everyone. I couldn't wait for Nick to wake up to show him.

It was a moment I realized that amid tragedy, and fear, and uncertainty—there could still be joy. We were aware of how peculiar and awful this moment in time was *and* of how special it was. There's always a silver lining, and for us, it was having this time to be siblings again, in a way we hadn't been in a long time.

Following the initial news story I did with *Good Morning America*, the news spread like wildfire. Press requests started flying in from every major news outlet. Diane Sawyer wanted to include the story in a feature she was doing on victims of the virus. *Entertainment Tonight* was preparing a big report. Gayle King reached out for an interview. Gayle King! I was in shock. I had written OPRAH'S RETREATS in giant letters across my vision board in January, and now I was one degree away from her. Outlets that couldn't get ahold of me directly started taking my Instagram posts and stories and publishing articles from them, embedding my profile in the text. Because of this, I woke up to thousands of new followers every day, thousands of new people to sing and dance with me. I had thousands of DMs from friends and strangers and celebrities. People were hearing the story and reaching out. They wanted to tell me to keep fighting, keep believing, keep singing. They also wanted to help.

A GoFundMe account had been started the day we learned about the amputation. I was texting with my friend and client Aimee Song, and she asked me if I had one. When I said no, she asked if she could set one up for me. Aimee has over five million followers on Instagram and a very successful business: when she starts something, it catches on. My friends Jacey Duprie, a famous LA lifestyle blogger whom I had begun training, and Erin Silver, the PR director for Volvo, joined to help her. These three new friends came together to rescue me. They knew I would need help. In the first twenty-four hours, it raised over $50,000 and kept growing.

I couldn't believe it every time I checked. Some people were giving $1,000, and some were giving $5, and all of those donations added up! You could scroll through the names and see them all, and I was completely overwhelmed with gratitude. So many people were out of work. So many people had to cancel vacations and weddings and take on unforeseen expenses. But they were giving what they could to a complete stranger. It brought me to tears. I had been worrying for weeks about Nick's medical bills and the additional home renovation costs now that we would have to make our little cottage accessible for him. This GoFundMe took away that huge fear and allowed me to breathe a little easier, knowing that at least I'd be able to afford whatever was coming our way. Every news outlet publicized it, friends shared it, and as I watched it continue to grow throughout the months ahead, I was in shock. It made me want to help others.

The deliveries, support, and love piled in that week. As the world learned this story, it felt like everyone wanted to do something to help.

Clients, friends, and PR companies that had my address on file sent gifts and goodies daily. The UPS man was our own personal Santa Claus. Every time we left and came back, we'd find new deliveries of flowers, groceries, or treats at the doorstep. Toys, clothes, and food for Elvis piled up; boxes regularly took over the cabin. Everything that arrived had to be sanitized, carefully unpacked, washed, sorted, and put away. Then the boxes had to be broken down and recycled. It took hours! You couldn't give anything away at this time because all the donation centers were closed because of COVID. But I gave what I could to friends who were helping. Each time a Stroller Buddy arrived to walk Elvis, they left with food, wine, workout clothes, and spa products.

"Thank you," we'd say, giving them a bouquet of flowers that had just arrived because we had nowhere to put it.

The whole Broadway community knew what had happened now and came to the rescue the way they knew best: with song.

Nick's cast from *Waitress* was the first to send me a video of the entire cast, along with composer-lyricist Sara Bareilles, singing "Live Your Life." They compiled all their voices singing different lines, and it was so thoughtful and beautiful that it brought me to tears.

This sparked a trend, and the next day I got a video from the cast of my first Broadway musical, *Good Vibrations*. The show had a Beach Boys theme, so the cast did a parody of "Wouldn't It Be Nice," in which they changed all the lyrics to be about Nick waking up and getting better.

Then the *Rock of Ages* cast sang us "Don't Stop Believing," and, finally, the *Jersey Boys* cast, after hearing "Can't Take My Eyes Off of You" was Elvis's favorite song, recorded an epic version of it. I've said it before, and I'll say it again: there's no people like show people. We are a tight-knit, loving, and expressive group, and they offered us support in the way Nick would have found most beautiful: through song.

Sarah Michelle Gellar got in touch with us through Instagram and asked if she could personally set up something called Meal Train for Todd, Anna, and me so we wouldn't have to worry about dinner anymore. It was a program where people could sign up to send us meals, and since figuring out dinner and cooking and cleaning had become a real burden, nightly deliveries were a huge relief. At the end of the night, we just wanted the work to be over and to be able to enjoy our evening together. This felt like a godsend. All we had to do was give her our address and phone number, and dinner started arriving at our door every night at seven thirty, just after we got Elvis down to bed. It was delivery from the best restaurants in the city: Sugarfish, Jon & Vinny's, California Chicken Cafe. Each meal was being provided by someone we didn't even know. It was incredible to realize people wanted to do this for us. We couldn't process what was happening. It was such a tremendous outpouring of love from the whole world in so many ways. None of it really made sense to me.

I reposted the stories of people singing and dancing with me every day and had begun to notice a few regulars. Tally Sessions, an actor friend we knew from Broadway shows, was always making up a skit and doing a full performance.

David Josefsberg, who dressed in a bedazzled Elvis costume, sang from a different location every day and with more enthusiasm than anyone.

My girlfriends Purdie Baumann, Lydia Holtz, and Allison Patterson never missed a single day of being there with me.

An entire family, the DeHopes, sang and danced every single day.

Even my neighbors in Laurel Canyon, just a few doors down—"I look forward to three p.m. all day long," Molly told me. "If I miss it, I'm devastated."

At Brown Bear, Anna was always there next to me, dancing, as was Elvis. We struggled daily to get the words right, but we sang anyway.

I started staying on after my Instagram Live at three to talk and give an update on Nick. It was becoming therapeutic, inspiring, and helpful to tune in every day and see this. There was a world united behind me, rooting for Nick to make it. It was hard to believe it was real. The more I shared, the more news channels picked up, and the further the story spread. Every day more articles were written, more people found out about us, followed along, and cheered and sang with me at three. #WakeUpNick had become a movement.

People weren't just singing with me; they were sending me articles, resources, and similar stories to inspire me or give me information. That was how I heard about Gregg Garfield.

Gregg was among the first people in the United States to get the virus. He caught it in January on an annual ski trip to Italy. His story was eerily similar to Nick's. He was fifty-three, perfectly healthy, and had no preexisting conditions. He wasn't that bad when he came into the emergency room, yet within less than forty-eight hours, he wasn't breathing well and was on maximum oxygen. He was intubated and on a ventilator for thirty-one days. His kidneys started failing, and his blood pressure plummeted. His lungs collapsed four times, he lost fingers and toes, and he was given a 1 percent chance of survival. His girlfriend, AJ, had been able to be in the hospital with him in the beginning because it was so early into the COVID scare that hospitals didn't have rules yet. Like me, she was FaceTiming Gregg and had no choice but to believe, during the darkest of times, that he would wake up. When he finally did, she was permitted to visit him at Burbank Hospital. Each hospital had different policies.

When I learned about them, I found their GoFundMe and donated to it.

They saw my donation, heard about me, and contacted me, offering to talk if I needed any support or information. It was incredible to talk to AJ. As she explained Gregg's story, the parallels to Nick's experience gave me hope that he, too, would wake up and recover just as Gregg had. AJ was so positive and reassuring and asked me a ton of questions that first night we spoke:

- What is his PEEP at?
- What was his heart rate today?
- What is his oxygen saturation rate?
- What are his vent settings?
- What was it yesterday?
- What medications is he on?

I couldn't answer most of them. I had no idea. Some of the things she said sounded familiar, but I wasn't sure what others meant at all.

Talking to AJ made me realize that I could ask and get more information, so I felt like I knew what was going on. She told me that I needed to call the hospital every day and ask these questions to the nurses. I needed this information so I could understand and track how he was progressing. I honestly still didn't know that I could ask these questions or that I was entitled to this information. I hadn't even met all of Nick's doctors, just Dr. Ng. Gregg was still in the hospital recovering when I spoke to AJ for the first time. She was allowed to visit him while he got strong enough to go home. Gregg's sister was there alongside her, helping. It was in so many ways the same story. Our conversation was so comforting because she knew exactly what I was going through, exactly how I felt.

AJ said to me, "Don't give up hope. We were just like you, staying positive, singing, and acting crazy in the house. We never once believed he wouldn't make it, even on the darkest days! We had an amazing doctor helping us through. I want to put you in touch with him—his name is John."

I called John immediately after AJ and I got off the phone. There was no time to waste, and I needed help. John has practiced medicine his entire adult life. He knows a lot of people, a lot about medicine, and a lot about Cedars-Sinai. From the second I talked to John, he became my medical advisor and friend. It was as if I had known him for years. I confided everything to him, Nick's whole story. "He's a beast, that husband of yours," he'd say.

John, who had never officially met me, took me on as a patient. He called and texted me every day, called doctors on my behalf, talked to anyone and everyone he possibly could to help me get into Cedars-Sinai or find ways to help Nick get better. One of the most helpful things was his translating what the doctors and nurses were telling me about Nick into a language I could understand, and then he would help me figure out what to ask them so we could stay on track or even get ahead of the game.

Nick had been slowly improving since the amputation—less assistance, clean CT scan results, fewer medications—and they were trying to take him off continuous dialysis. Things were looking up. But everything can change in the ICU in an instant, throwing all the progress just made right out the window. Over the next few days, that's precisely what happened.

On the morning of April 24, I was just about to sit down to a fluffy stack of pancakes Anna had made for me when the phone rang. It was the hospital.

"He had a little bit of an eventful night. He's been having these episodes anytime he gets moved or repositioned where his heart rate suddenly drops really low. This has been happening, but last night, there was one moment when his heart kinda paused for close to twenty seconds, and honestly—that's pretty long. These are becoming much more frequent, so we've had the cardiologist look at him, and we decided he's going to need some temporary pacing wires; little wires that, if his heart rate drops, a pacemaker will be able to take over for him."

Dr. Ng told me to think of the heart like a house. There are plumbing and electrical systems involved in running the heart. Nick's overall heart functions were great, the plumbing was working—pumping—but his electrical system needed some help.

It was a relief to hear that, and this news was delivered so calmly and routinely, it didn't alarm me. But the call ended with "We also need to put him back on continuous dialysis, and his vent settings are going to need just a touch more help—just a touch."

That was crushing; all the progress we had just made with those things was now undone. *A pacemaker?* It was another thing, another machine. I hated hearing about these irregular heart rates and wondered if they were a result of his being on hydroxychloroquine. Trying to figure out what caused what through every step of this drove me mad. I gave my consent a moment later when the nurse called.

Dr. Ng assured me this wasn't a big backward step; it was more like a sideways step. It was just to help keep him stable. Stable was good.

The next day the pacemaker was safely in and working.

I couldn't see a real physical difference, just an added silver plate on the left side of his neck connected to more wires. They were trying to schedule the tracheostomy and put in a feeding tube to get Nick more calories, but those had to wait. While they told me this wasn't really a setback, in my mind it was. He was back on continual dialysis, and he was on another machine. The MRI still hadn't been done, and we had no more insight into when he would wake up.

I had learned by now that the nurses switched shifts at seven a.m., so to get the overnight news about Nick, I could call around six thirty.

Unfortunately, when I called the morning of April 25, the report was not good. Nick had had a bad night. Completely out of nowhere, he had spiked a fever. That caused his blood pressure to drop, and they had to put him back on the highest dose of blood pressure medication. The feeding tube and trach were now on the back burner—the new focus was to find the source of this fever.

They were going to go deep into his lungs and take a look with a bronchoscope, and get samples to test for COVID again, as well as for any and every other infection that could possibly be causing a fever. It was crucial to find the cause and treat it. When a patient is critical, the body is so weak and stressed that a tiny infection could result in death.

The bronchoscope procedure found an infection deep in his lungs that had been there, untreated, for a while. It went into his blood, which caused him to go into septic shock.

"Septic shock" were two words I had heard about before. This can happen from being in the hospital for too long. I knew it wasn't good.

Dr. Ng told me there were planning a bronchial sweep, which he referred to as a "bronch." They would be calling for my consent, but I had no idea what it was. So like everything, the moment the call ended, I got on Google. I learned that it's the equivalent of a power wash for your lungs. Another doctor called me to explain further what a bronch sweep was. They were going to go through Nick's mouth, down the esophagus, and deep into his lungs to suction out all the mucus from the infection. Then they test samples of the mucus to determine what kind of infection he had so they could treat it more effectively.

Afterward, Nick was put on the most potent antibiotic the hospital had to try to kill this infection. It could be administered for only seven days, and we would know within the first forty-eight hours or so if it was helping. We just had to wait—another waiting game to play.

Following a rough couple of days, Nick seemed to be getting back on track by the afternoon of April 28. The antibiotics were helping, and they were weaning him off the blood pressure medications again. I got a call from Debra, a social worker at Cedars-Sinai, that morning. I hadn't been allowed to visit for the past two days, but she said that I could come to the hospital for an official meeting with the doctors. It was time for me to sit down with Nick's team and hear what was going on from them directly, she explained.

I was finally allowed back in, and I felt like meeting with the whole team would give me some real clarity. After the meeting, I would be able to spend an hour with Nick.

I immediately called Dr. John, who was elated; after all, he had been on the phone for weeks trying to get through to someone. It seemed like his efforts, and my persistence, had finally paid off. I walked into Saperstein that day, not really knowing what to expect. I was eager to meet the doctors and finally put some faces to names, but I was also a little nervous. Every time I stepped into the hospital, things felt much more real and scarier.

Debra met me when I got off the elevator and escorted me to a small meeting room on Nick's floor. I glanced into Nick's room as I walked by. In the meeting room were the ICU doctors, Dr. Ng, and Nick's nurse for the day. The ICU doctors rotate every two weeks, so I met Dr. Adrian Williams and Dr. Julian Welch, who had been on Nick's case and had treated him.

The room had concrete walls and no windows. It consisted only of a table and several mismatched chairs. Bright, fluorescent lights beamed down on us from the ceiling. The room looked like it hadn't been used in years. It was cold and uninviting.

We sat down at the table—I was on one side and the Cedars-Sinai medical team was on the other. It felt like I was auditioning for a part in a show. I was determined to be strong, to react calmly, and to be confident. I had never had a meeting like this and didn't know what was going to happen. But I knew I had to control myself and learn. At this point, I hadn't talked to the other doctors, only to Dr. Ng.

They welcomed me and started by apologizing for how hard this must be for me. They said how hard it was for them and for the nurses.

"This isn't normal; everything is different," they said, especially for them.

Right off the bat, I learned some eye-opening things. In normal times, I could have been at the hospital every day; I could have slept there if I wanted. In normal times, I would have met Nick's team on day one and would have talked to them every day. In normal times, I would have been a part of everything, attended all the meetings, with nothing off-limits. But these were not normal times.

They gave me a recap of everything that had happened since Nick entered the ICU.

Dr. Williams had performed the surgery to put Nick on ECMO. Apparently, Nick was so critical after ECMO that they didn't think he would make it through the night.

He had three towers of medicines just to keep him alive.

Dr. Welch had been doing Nick's bronchial sweeps since the infections had gotten worse. Nick's lungs weren't looking great. COVID and his pneumonia had done severe damage to them. These were all big problems, but the biggest, overlying issue was that he wasn't waking up. They all needed him to wake up. It was taking a long time, too long. It was starting to get worrisome.

Dr. Ng and I had been remaining positive, but ICU doctors see critical patients every day. This meeting was the first time I understood how everyone's outlook is much grimmer in the ICU. It's not to say they aren't lovely people; it's just a critical atmosphere all the time. Death is something they are used to. It's inevitably what they witness day in and day out, so they don't really sugarcoat things. I hadn't talked to them before—I was used to the sugar and the upside from my optimistic doctor. This other outlook was a lot to hear and process. I felt baffled.

Debra sat and listened, and Nick's nurse only chimed in with little bits of information here and there. I was in shock as they spoke and I wanted to scream—but I didn't. I didn't cry. I didn't get frustrated. I didn't raise my voice. I sat there holding my ground, asking whatever questions I could think of.

At the end of the meeting, I got up and said, "If you want my husband to wake up, then you need to let me in this hospital every day. I know that it's not up to you. But whoever isn't letting me visit needs to be spoken to. I have talked to so many people who say how important it is to have your loved one next to you when you're in a coma. They need to hear and feel you. Nick *needs* me by his side. You have to let me back in!"

They all nodded while I spoke. They heard me and agreed. They agreed, but it wasn't their choice. They promised to try to help, to do their best to get me access.

Debra led me to Nick's room after the meeting was over and said she would see what she could do. If there was anything else she could help with, I was to let her know. It finally dawned on me why I needed a social worker for this. Debra was there to *help* me, to make sure I was okay. To make sure I was emotionally stable. She could speak for me. I thought back to when she first called. I had wondered why in the world this woman was calling me, thinking I didn't need her. But maybe I *did* need a Debra.

I got to Nick's room and ran to his side. He was lying in his bed, all alone in this quiet room. I wanted to scream, to release the emotions that had built up during the meeting. But I remained strong—for him. I grabbed his hand in mine and kissed his forehead. I started rubbing his head.

"Nick, I just had a big meeting with all your doctors! You are going to be just fine, babe!"

He didn't need to know what I had just been told.

"We gotta get this infection cleared up and your lungs clean, but other than that, you are doing great! We need you to wake up, though. You've got to wake up, Nick! Your name is Nick Cordero . . ."

And I went through the rest of my script.

They gave me an hour with him, and then I was told to leave. I left the music on for him and asked his nurse to make sure it kept playing before profusely thanking her for being amazing and caring for my husband. I was beyond grateful for any time I could have. Debra told me to call in the morning to see if I could come back, so at least I left there with a little hope.

As soon as I got out to the street, I broke down into tears. Being strong for that long felt like I had been holding my breath underwater for twenty minutes. I got to my car and just sat in the seat, frozen and unable to drive. I decided to call Lesley and fill her in on the meeting. Lesley was always so supportive of whatever I was doing in the hospital and was grateful that they had let me in. Once off the phone, I just sat there, unable to bring myself to start the car. I sat thinking about Nick, how he couldn't wake up. How if, and when, he woke up, he wouldn't have a leg. I thought about how weak he was, how thin he had become. It was devastating. It made me feel so grateful that I could move, and it instantly made me think of the question I always get asked about fitness. *How do you stay motivated on days you just don't want to work out?*

After this long afternoon, after seeing Nick's leg again, and after hearing how sick my husband was, I decided to go on Instagram and share my thoughts.

We are so lucky to be able to wake up, to stand on two feet, to walk, to jump, to skip, and to smile. Do not ever take that for granted! If you have ever been injured or know someone who can't physically move, you know how lucky you are to be able to move your body! Do not take it for granted!! Use your body, strengthen your body, take care of your body! Be grateful! I know that if Nick was awake, all he would want to do is get up and go for a walk, play with Elvis, or work out. You can do it! Do it for Nick! Do it for the COVID patients around the world who are lying in hospital beds on ventilators. Move your body!

When I got back to Brown Bear, I sat at the table with Todd and Anna and told them how the meeting had gone. I told them how the doctors had just stared at me as they delivered this news, how Debra had talked to me in a hushed tone, and how they all had treated me as if, at any moment, I was going to shatter.

Anna and Todd never knew what to say. No one did. But it was a relief to have people to come home to and talk to, people to whom I could relay what had happened. I didn't want to be hugged; I felt claustrophobic. I just wanted to cry to people who loved me.

"I think it's so good, sister," Anna said, "that you stayed so strong in there. That you didn't cry or yell. They were probably expecting you to. They probably were waiting for it. I'm sure most people who receive news like that lose it! You're fighting this battle with them to let you in the door and let you be by his side—and tonight you proved that you can take it. You can take the bad news and remain calm, and strong, and hopeful."

I suddenly felt pride as I realized what I had done instinctively. I had shown them I was strong, and calm, and a fighter—just like Nick. It was a daily battle to be allowed in the hospital, and I still didn't understand why. Nick had been deemed critical, which meant I should be allowed to visit. But the rules continued to change every day, adding to the roller coaster of emotions I already felt. My only theory as to *why* was that some people there thought I was crazy, unstable. But I had shown them—after they threw all their worst news at me and shared their doomed outlook—that I could sit there, digest it all, and say, "Okay, so what do we need to do to fix this?"

"These aren't normal times," they kept reiterating. But I had shown them I could take it. I had shown them that I was not a normal woman.

ten

Everyone had warned me that the ICU is a roller coaster. They said there would be ups and downs, highs and lows, adrenaline rushes, and moments so awful you have to cover your eyes.

Two hours from where I grew up in Ohio is America's biggest theme park, Cedar Point. It boasts seventeen coasters, each with a different accolade: fastest, tallest, greatest number of inversions. I grew up going every summer with my family, every Memorial Day weekend after the prom, and every Halloween with a group of friends for Fright Fest. I'm a veteran coaster rider.

But nothing can prepare you for the actual ride that is the ICU, the twists and turns in the track that you don't see coming. There are moments when you have cranked to the top of the hill and feel invincible, and then a sudden, speeding plummet makes you lose your stomach. There are times when you smile because you just survived what seemed impossible, and times when you are so scared you want to scream. There are moments when you throw your hands into the air and surrender to falling, and other times when you grab the sides of the car as tight as you possibly can because you are so terrified. Some parts of the track seem to happen in slow motion, but overall the ride is going so fast you don't have time to process your reactions before it suddenly comes to a screeching stop. You just have to hope it ends the way it's supposed to: with you and your partner getting up and walking off, saying, "That was a wild ride—but we survived it."

I was allowed back into the hospital the next day in the late afternoon. Debra had come through, it seemed. Todd and Anna stayed with Elvis, and I drove myself. The timing of the visits had become so erratic that it was easier for me to drive myself, allowing Todd to focus on getting work done. I went into Nick's room and found him the same way I'd left him the night before: alone and asleep. I did my usual speech, my usual routine, and then I told him stories about Elvis. He was getting so big, changing every day. In my absence, he had really come around to Anna. Todd was trying to get back to work after having taken the last three weeks off, so Anna was taking over as Elvis's stand-in mom. Little ak! was back in action as my substitute yet again.

Elvis was crawling all over the house now—fascinated by buckles, zippers, and drawers. Yesterday he had opened all the drawers in the kitchen and emptied everything out of all of them onto the kitchen floor. I came out to find Anna sitting on the floor in the middle of the mess as he was throwing an entire pack of Ziploc bags around. I looked at her, stunned, and she said, "Don't worry, I'm watching. I just figured that he's going to do this whether I stop him or not, so I'm letting him make the disaster because it keeps him happy and entertained, and then I'll clean it all up."

I told him about how cute Todd was with Elvis. How he had gone to Target and come back with a whole new wardrobe for him because it was getting so warm and he had no shorts. I told him how his cast from *Rock of Ages* was saving us with the daily walks. I imitated Zoe, who, the second she got the stroller in her hands, would start singing "Old McDonald had a farm," in an operatic tone with her thick, Australian accent, while Elvis screamed because he was being taken away from us. I told him how we had all made dinner together with vegetables

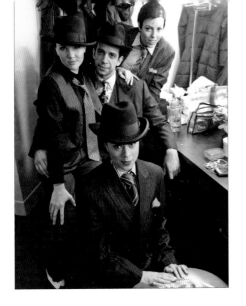

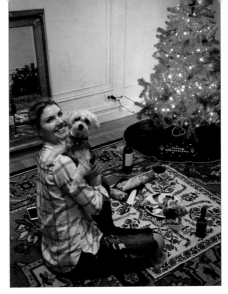

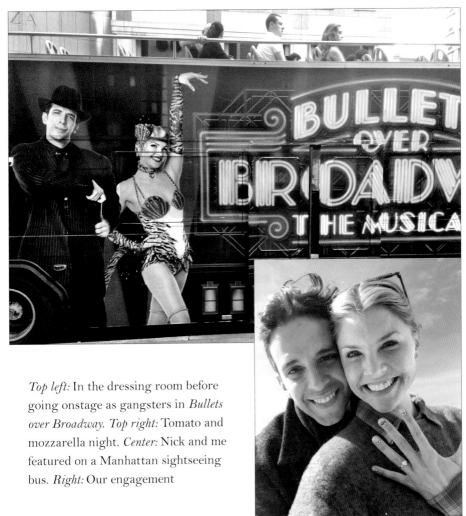

Top left: In the dressing room before going onstage as gangsters in *Bullets over Broadway. Top right:* Tomato and mozzarella night. *Center:* Nick and me featured on a Manhattan sightseeing bus. *Right:* Our engagement

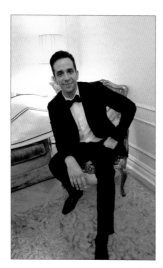

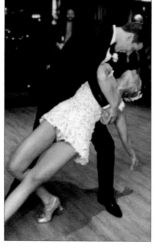

Far left: Nick before our wedding
Left: Our wedding dance
(Photo by Andrew Holtz)

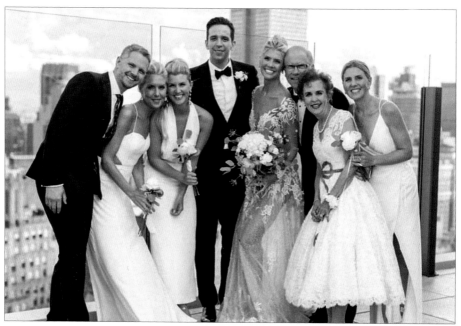

Nick becoming a Kloots *(Photo by Andrew Holtz)*

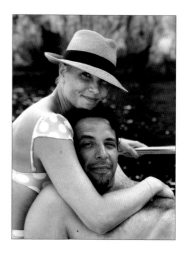

Phase 1 of our honeymoon: Capri

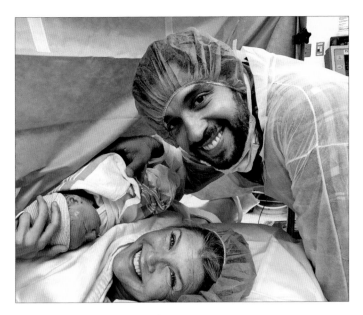

Minutes after Elvis was born

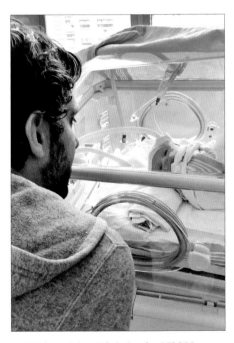

Nick visiting Elvis in the NICU

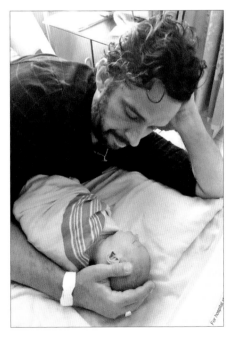

New dad

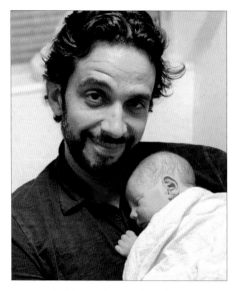

Nick holding Elvis on his chest

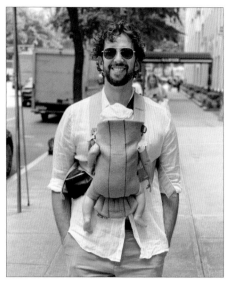

New York City dad

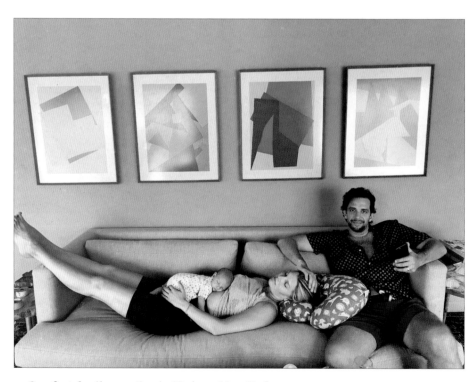

Our first family vacation in Hudson, New York

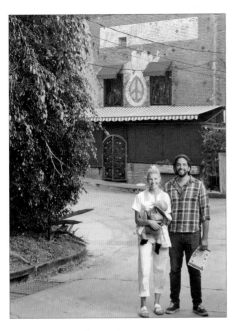

Moments after going to our open house

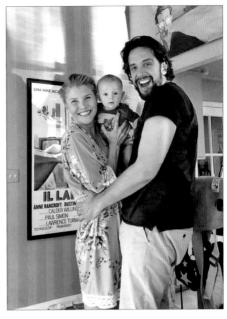

Moments after finding out we got the house

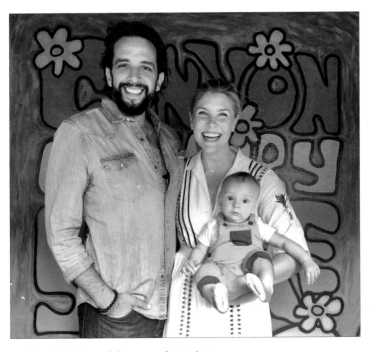

Our first Laurel Canyon photo day

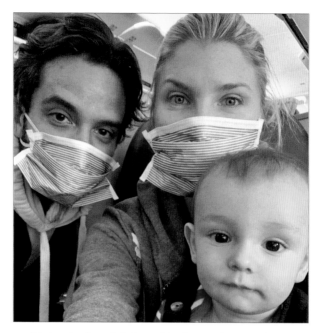

Flying back to LA from Manhattan in March 2020

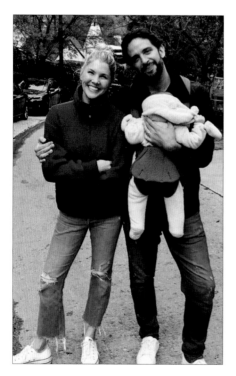

My birthday, March 19, 2020

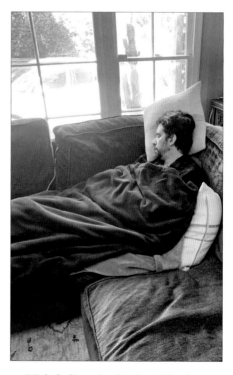

Nick feeling tired in late March

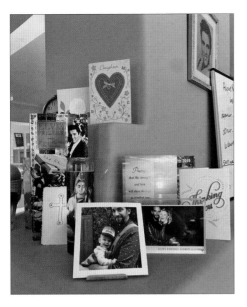

Our "Wake Up Nick" display

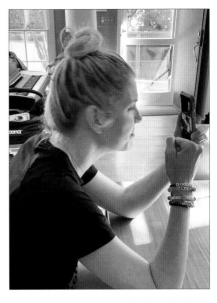

Facetiming Nick in the hospital

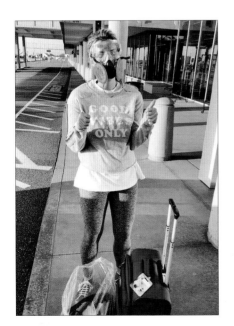

Anna on her way to LA

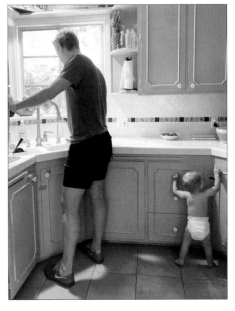

Elvis getting into mischief while Todd cleans

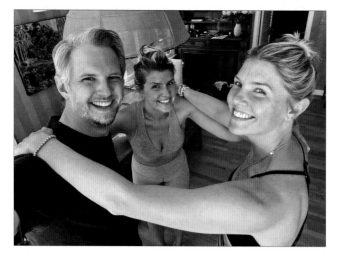

Left: The new circle
Center left: Sleeping next to my phone in case the doctor calls
Center right: Todd explains the "secrecy of the sisters"

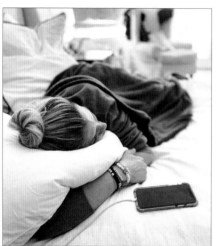

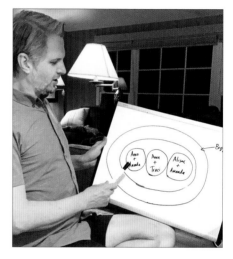

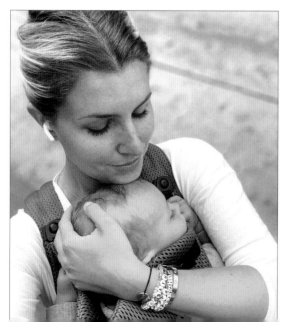

Anna taking Elvis on a Canyon walk

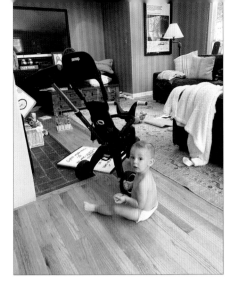

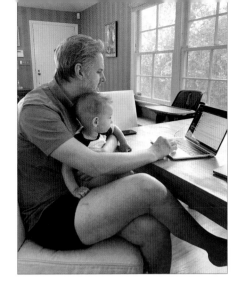

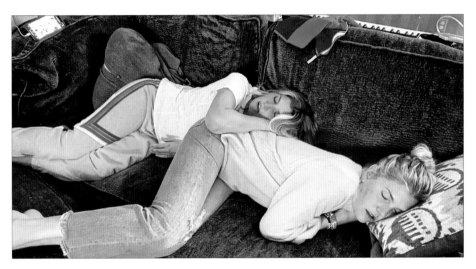

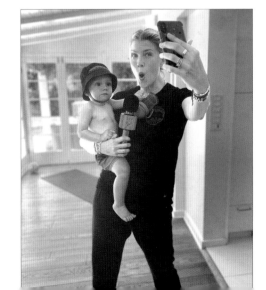

Top left: The general state of the cabin. *Top right:* Trying to balance work and babies
Center: Nightly exhaustion
Right: Going live at 3 PM

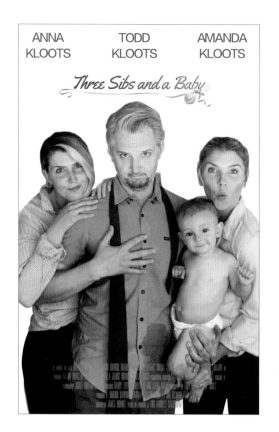

Our homemade movie poster for *Three Sibs and a Baby*

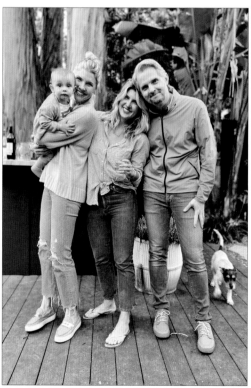

The quaranteam

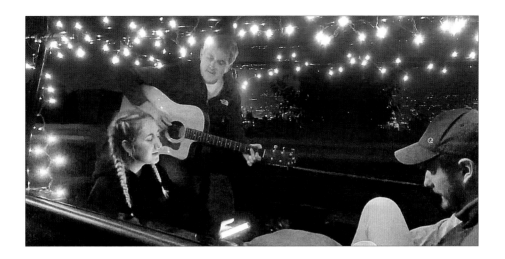

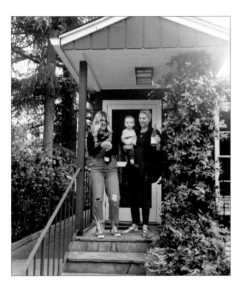

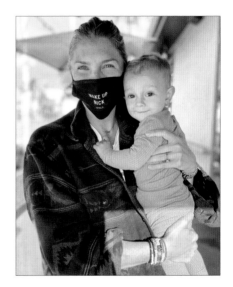

Top left: Jono's twinkle-lit truck
with Lenii singing
Center left: Popping champagne
outside Brown Bear after the news
that Nick is awake
Center right: Coffee run with
Elvis. *Right:* Celebrating at
Sunday choir that Nick is awake

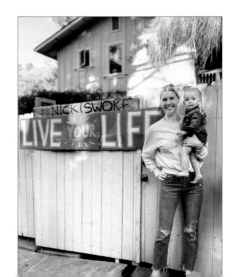

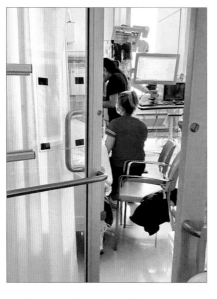

Visiting Nick in late May

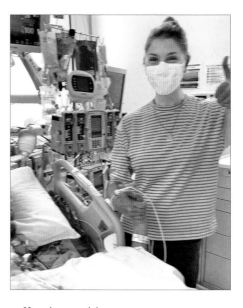

Keeping positive

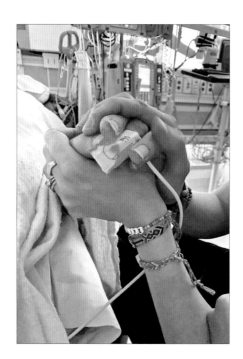

Finally holding Nick's hand

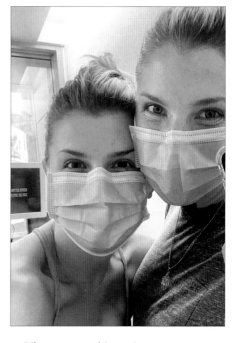

The pep squad in action

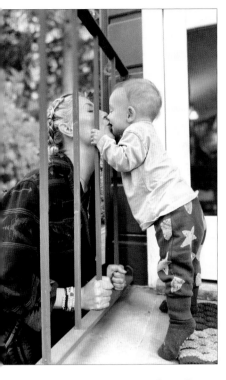

Kisses for Mama on Mother's Day

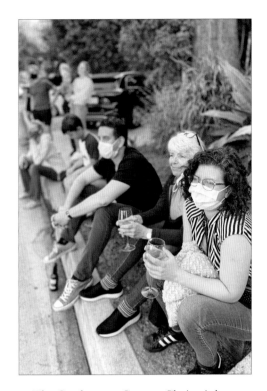

The Corderos at Canyon Choir night

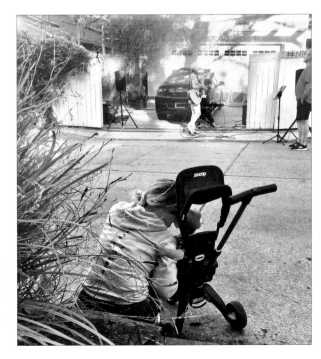

Anna and Elvis, the
founding members
of the Laurel Canyon
Community Choir

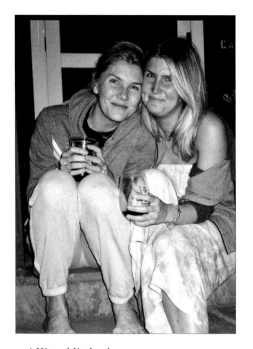

AK! and little ak

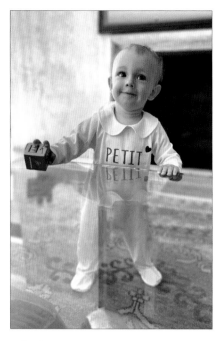

Petit

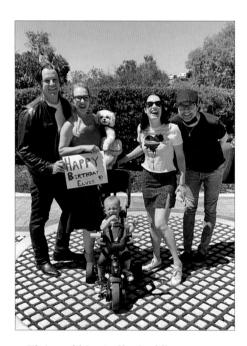

Elvis and his stroller buddies

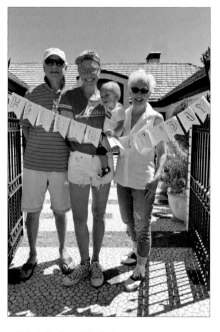

Elvis's first birthday

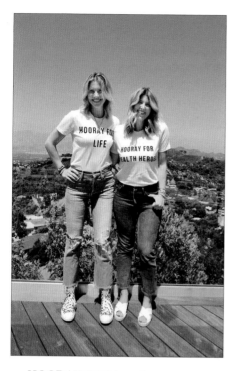

HOORAY FOR launch

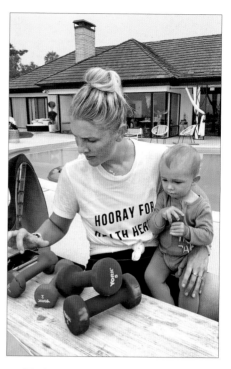

Trying to do it all

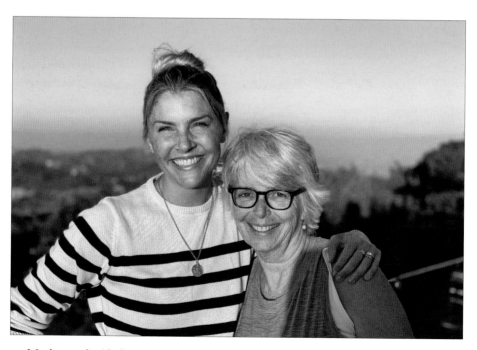

Mother and wife dream team

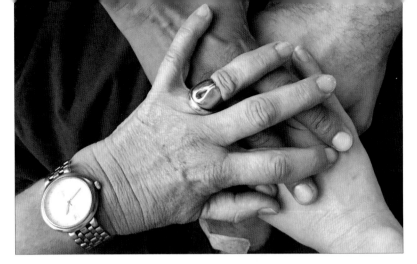

Above: The
Corderos hold
hands with Eduardo
one last time
Right: Elvis and I
hold hands with Nick
one last time

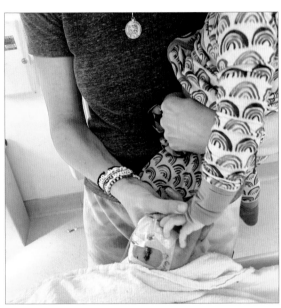

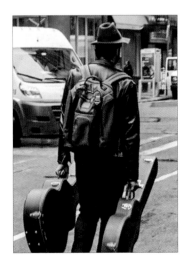

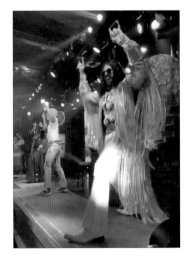

Far left: Nick
headed to the
studio
Left: Nick
in the finale
of *Rock of
Ages,* 2020

from Zach's garden the night before and how at midnight Anna had ordered us five pints of Salt & Straw because she could tell I needed a little pick-me-up.

I was getting ready to leave when Dr. Welch came into the room. He had heard I was visiting and wanted to talk to me. The bronch that morning had startled him, he said. He took me into the little anteroom outside Nick's—the one where I had stood on the day of the amputation. He had Nick's CT scans with him. "Has anyone showed you these?" he asked. He took me over to the computer and opened Nick's file.

He wasn't trying to scare me, but as we sat there, alone in that small room, he delivered a heavy dose of reality, and it was horrifying.

"Look," he said, showing me the scans. I cried and asked what this meant for Nick's life. "If it were my wife in there, I'd want to keep fighting, too. Nick is young. If he was seventy, this would be a different story. But he's young. So we fight."

I was defeated. It was truly the first time that I felt like Nick might not make it, that what I was doing was useless. I called Lesley when I got to my car that night. I needed to vent, to tell someone the new harsh reality I had just heard. It was so out of left field to both of us—that even as I was recounting it all, it didn't sound real. But the problem was, it *was* real. I had seen the evidence: the scans, the massive holes in his lungs. I understood why the infection wasn't getting better and couldn't get better. I relayed the news to Lesley because she needed to know.

It was dark by the time I pulled into the driveway of the cabin. I could see the scene through the screen door. Todd and Anna were arranging food on the table and setting down plates. Dinner was ready. I hadn't been at the hospital this late before. They knew that radio silence for hours was probably not good news—but rather than panic, they had taken action.

Brown Bear, which I had left in a disastrous state that morning, was now spotless. I should be walking in to a hungry, exhausted toddler and all the dishes from the day, but with Bibbidi-Bobbidi and Biggie, that was never the case. There was a candle burning and a fresh vase of sunflowers on the table. They had bathed Elvis and put him to bed. They had ordered carbs. A lot of carbs.

Todd and Anna knew from the way I walked in the door that my visit had not gone well, but instead of pressing me for details, my sister simply handed me a glass of red wine.

I wish I was one of those people who can't eat during trauma, but I'm the opposite. I left the hospital feeling so drained, so exhausted, that coming home to a feast of carbohydrates and good wine kept me going. I sat down and grabbed a piece of sourdough and chewed while they gave me the highlights of my son's day.

I always felt consumed with both gratitude and sadness as they told their anecdotes. It was already hard that Nick was missing his son growing up, but every time I spent an entire day at the hospital, I felt I was missing it, too. But at the same time, watching the bond Elvis was forming with Todd and Anna warmed my heart. My siblings are my best friends—they always have been. When you have a child, you want him to know and love all the people you love most. Under normal circumstances, they're scattered all over the world, but during these strange, unforeseen times, at least, the three of us were together.

I took a deep breath, and then shared what had happened at the hospital.

"Dr. Welch told me Nick's lungs look like someone who's been smoking ten packs a day for fifty years. They have holes—enormous holes—that will never heal. There is so much bacteria and infection that he is not improving, despite the heavy antibiotics he's on.

"He said if he lives through this, he'll probably carry around oxygen for the rest of his life.

"He said if he lives through this, he might be in a wheelchair for the rest of his life.

"He believes there's a good chance that if he does wake up, his speech will be drastically affected.

"He may never be able to move his arms normally again because of where the strokes occurred.

"He may not be able to chew.

"He may not be able to move the right side of his body.

"But even in the best-case scenario, Dr. Welch is confident that because of the damage to his lungs, Nick will never live a normal life."

I delivered my monologue in monotone, looking down at my plate and repeatedly poking a noodle with my fork.

I had sat through this conversation just an hour before and was still trying to process it, to decide if it was real. Dr. Ng was my "positive doctor"; tonight Dr. Welch earned the reputation of "bearer of bad news." As the doctor delivered these life-altering blows, I watched Nick through the window, just lying there, his face barely visible under a mess of tubes.

To make things worse, he told me Nick was back in a state of sepsis, which happens when an infection you already have triggers a chain reaction throughout your body and rapidly leads to tissue damage, organ failure, and often death. I knew this from my research after his last bout of sepsis; I understood it was bad. It's what had caused him to briefly die on the table a month before.

This time last night, everything looked good. His amputation was healing well, his blood pressure was down, and they were going to take him off the ventilator. Today was the first time I understood the true extent of the damage COVID had done, understood that my husband would not make a full recovery and live a normal life. Nor would we.

"I just don't understand why," I cried.

It was the question I asked myself every night: *Why is this happening to my husband?*

It made no sense. He was so young, and he had his whole life to live, and he was healthy. All he had ever wanted was to live in Laurel Canyon, be a father, have his child go to Wonderland, perform his music. It was unbearable for me, as his wife, to go through the day knowing he was lying there alone, fighting, instead of enjoying what he had worked so hard to have. I didn't understand it.

My siblings went quiet because they didn't either.

Our silence was broken by the sound of a car pulling into the driveway.

"Who's here?" I asked, wiping my eyes on the collar of Nick's flannel I was wearing. I was slowly taking over his belongings, looking for any way to have a piece of him with me.

"This may sound like the worst idea right now, but I think it's exactly what you need," Anna said. "Jono is here—let's go outside."

The young Irish singer Lenii and her bandmates were still staying with my neighbor Jono. He was trying to help her launch her career, and they figured there was no better time to work on an album than when you're forced to stay inside. It was them in the driveway: Jono in the driver's seat and the whole band, complete with a keyboard, violin, and guitar in the bed of a black pickup truck, which was decorated in twinkle lights.

We sat on the steps of Brown Bear on the chilly spring night.

"We came to sing you a song," Jono said.

This hurts like hell, but it feels right . . .

While the band played and the lights flickered, Lenii sang a slow, acoustic version of "Live Your Life" that still haunts me. Anna, Todd, and I huddled close together on the stone steps outside the guesthouse, silently crying, our arms wrapped around one another.

But it's all right, live your life.
Like you've got one night, live your life.
Yes, it's all right, live your life.

Like you've got one night, live your life.
They'll give you hell—but don't you let them kill your light, not with-
  out a fight.

This moment was precisely why Nick had wanted to live in Laurel Canyon. The community, the music. This scene was right out of a movie; you couldn't have written it more perfectly. In what world does a truck, covered in twinkle lights, show up in your driveway with musicians to serenade you with a live acoustic version of your husband's song? These things don't happen.

But it's normal here—on Lookout Mountain, this is normal. Nick knew that, and at this moment, I knew I was so lucky to be here, with this community supporting me.

With moments like that one, I believed we would get our miracle, our Code Rocky. Even on days like that one, when I felt so defeated and so frustrated. I got angry—but then I prayed, and believed, and stayed positive that my husband would make it home.

I kept fighting.

eleven

The only reason I slept that night was because of my full belly and half a Xanax. I fell asleep, yet again, with my phone in my hand, hoping and praying that it wouldn't ring in the middle of the night. I was so drained mentally and emotionally that I just allowed myself to shut down.

I called Dr. Ng as soon as I woke up the next morning. I needed my positive doctor. He had never brought up this lung damage, and I wanted him to explain it to me. I told him about seeing the scans and what Dr. Welch had said about Nick's lungs being destroyed.

"Doctor," I said, "he made it sound like Nick had no chance, like this damage was too severe to recover from."

"No," he said, "it's not. We definitely don't want it to get worse; we need to make sure we get the secretions out with daily bronch sweeps and keep them clean—but it's okay. Those things are going to heal. He has probably lost some lung function, but my general inclination is that his lungs *look* much more concerning than the function will show. Time will tell—but I've seen this often. Time will heal it."

On the other end of the phone, I couldn't get words out.

"I . . . uh . . . so you're telling me . . . um . . . Dr. Welch made it seem so bad last night, but now you're saying I don't need to be so scared? Why did Welch think it was severe damage?"

Dr. Ng explained, "He's mainly in the ICU, so he sees patients only in the critical state, not as they heal up. I see people who have bleak outlooks in the ICU and also as they recover. I share his concern, but for me—those are things that will improve. We don't know the fallout; we don't know what will happen. But I see people all the time who improve. We don't know if he's going to fall into that bucket—but why not?"

What I had been terrified about the night before now seemed unimportant. How could there be such a drastic difference in the outlook of two top doctors? It was scary because I didn't know which one to believe.

The last thing Dr. Ng had said was: "Amanda, it's confusing stuff—it's not like anyone is right or wrong. It's just different opinions. God gave us a lot more lung than we need. I think he can function like this. What his limitations will be, I can't tell you yet. But he is improving, and I expect him to heal well."

I hung up the phone and talked it through with Todd and Anna. They had been listening to the call, too, and were just as confused as I was. I had been counting Nick out when I went to sleep, but now I felt like there was hope, like he could be completely okay. I had spent the entire night sobbing and devastated and trying to come to terms with the inevitability Dr. Welch had described. Now I was smiling again; things seemed all right. But I was afraid to trust it. How could two doctors, both at the top of their field, have such different outlooks? I wanted to believe Dr. Ng, my optimistic doctor. But what if he wasn't right?

Even though I had just woken up, I was exhausted.

After breakfast, I curled up on my bed and took a nap, my phone inches from my face.

I came out to find Anna dancing around the kitchen with Elvis, who was in his carrier. She was blasting the soundtrack from *Tangled*, sweeping the floor, and feeding Elvis puffs. There was banana bread baking in the oven, and the kitchen was sparkling clean.

Todd was trying to get some work done, so she was on duty. But soon after I woke up, they did a handoff, and Elvis sat on Todd's lap while he reviewed some possible layouts for the new bathroom in our house. We were having to change everything to make it accessible for Nick. I cut a slice of warm banana bread and thanked God for my siblings.

Todd and Anna had asked everyone on the Code Rocky group to give me space that day, and I really appreciated it. It was hard to ask for silence—but when I got the courage to do it, I realized how much I needed it. For a solid month, my phone, email, and doorstep had become Grand Central Station. Deliveries never stopped coming; my phone was always ringing, beeping, or buzzing. My in-box was flooded with messages, and my DMs were out of control. I was so amazed and grateful for how invested everyone was; it made me feel encouraged to see everyone fighting with us. But the messages had become stressful, too, and when I wasn't answering them, I was trying to research things for Nick. I couldn't put my devices down. I couldn't miss a call. I couldn't risk leaving a message unread—what if it contained something important? I couldn't not respond to friends and family when they checked in with me—even though I knew they would understand—it felt rude.

Before I went to bed that night, I took the whiteboard we had been using for notes, quotes, and grocery lists; erased the scribbles; and wrote, in big bold letters: "Miracle May." A new month felt like a fresh start. Nick's mom had been working with a healer who had assured her May was when Nick was going to wake up. Anna had a feeling, too. She kept saying he would wake up on Mother's Day as the ultimate gift to me.

I lay on the couch next to Todd, with my head in Anna's lap, and thought about everything that had happened over the last month, and it seemed impossible that so much could have happened in such a short time. It felt like a year's worth of events, not just thirty days. I tried to tell myself we had made it through that first month, still strong and standing. We would make it through another. We would get our miracle, and Nick would wake up this month and be home in time for Elvis's birthday in June.

To start our new month on a positive note, we planned to go to the beach the next day. A friend had graciously offered me her bungalow on a private stretch of the beach in Malibu any time I wanted it. I am a true Pisces; I am in my element around the water, so the ocean is always a healing place for me. Elvis didn't want to put even his toes in, but Anna and I soaked up as much vitamin sea as possible.

I had been allowed into the hospital that morning because at 3:15 that afternoon, Nick was getting his tracheostomy and having a feeding tube put in. These two procedures were something that we had been trying to get done for weeks. Since they were considered a "surgery," they made a case for me to visit and give my consent. The tracheostomy would make Nick more comfortable, get everything off his face, and make bronchial sweeps easier on him. The feeding tube would be helpful in administering medications and also getting more nourishment into him.

We took a long walk down the beach, which was bizarre because it was empty. It was nice to just walk and think and be outside by the water. Walking through Laurel Canyon is a million hills; it was nice to be on flat sand and far from the guesthouse, where it felt like the world was constantly coming down on us.

At five p.m., I received the call saying he made it through the surgery. He was on the trach and a feeding tube. He got a G-tube, to be exact. It connects right to his stomach so liquid food can go right into his system. It was a huge relief. Nick was so fragile; every time they did anything, it was cause for concern.

I woke up the next morning to positive messages from all over the world: Brazil, India, Romania, Scotland, Ireland, France, Spain, Mexico, Australia, Wales, London, Singapore, Guatemala, Honduras, Cyprus, Belgium, Bosnia, Budapest, Montenegro, Switzerland, and Russia.

My positive thought of the day instantly came to mind.

"He's got the whole world in his hands!"

This used to be one of my favorite songs to sing during Sunday school and also at night before I went to bed. As a little girl, I was scared of the dark, and if I couldn't sleep, I would lie on my belly and bounce my forehead to my pillow, singing my favorite church songs. I knew that singing songs about Jesus would comfort me and make me forget that I was scared.

He's got the whole world in his hands. He's got the whole wide world, in his hands. He's got the whole world in his hands. He's got the whole world in his hands.

Our story had reached the whole world, and people from all over the world were with me, supporting and praying for us. God had us in His hands.

I wanted to thank everyone for their support, prayers, and love, so I did what I knew best: exercised. I knew how many people were home with no way to work out, so I led a free workout on Instagram so people in quarantine could get moving. As a teacher, a trainer, I love sharing workouts to encourage anyone to get up and go. I was so inspired by everyone that I wanted to do what I could to give back.

I was on a high after class. Nick was doing well, I had a flood of support, and I had just finished a workout. I called the hospital to see when I could come in that day. But the call did not go as I had hoped.

"Unfortunately," I was told, "they aren't allowing you to come in today, or at all, until further notice."

They didn't think that I was following the Safer at Home order and taking quarantine rules seriously. They saw on my Instagram that I was "leading fitness classes" and hanging around my sister and friends. It took all my energy not to explode. Nick needed me! I needed him. I wasn't doing anything wrong. I was confused and heartbroken. I called Debra immediately to explain, hoping that she could help relay the truth to the nurses.

The fitness classes were done live online so people could join from their homes. I was not with them. My sister and brother lived with me and have been living with me for weeks. We were all completely isolated and safe. If anyone was following the rules, trust me, it was *me*! Debra told me I would be getting a call soon from the ICU director to explain.

I picked up the line, trying my best to remain calm as he and the head nurse on Nick's floor told me that with COVID, visiting was too risky and the special treatment they had been giving me was unfair. Some families had never been allowed to see their loved ones; they simply couldn't let me visit every day. Now that I was becoming recognizable in the media, I think their concerns doubled that I would be recognized entering or leaving the hospital. Word that they were "breaking the rules" for me would get out. I knew this was true, and they were right. But it was a hard pill to swallow, and I still fought back. Nick needed me; I *knew* it. I knew if I was in there, he would improve. They had witnessed the results of that; his numbers got better during my visits. Couldn't this be part of the treatment? I knew it was unconventional, but so what? There is only so much medicine can do at a certain point, and then the power of love kicks in. But they were not giving in. The only way I could get back in to see Nick was if he once again became critical and they thought he would likely die. What a thing to hear! "The next time I'll be able to visit is when you think he's going to *die*," I pleaded.

This was May. There was still so little known about the virus, and I understand now the hospital administration was just doing its best to keep themselves, the doctors, nurses, and other patients safe. Now we know so much more about the virus, how it spreads, the actual risks. They were making decisions based on what they knew at the time, but the consequence of those decisions was heartbreaking for me.

The report the next morning was that his vent settings were down, which was a great sign. We were always hoping for less assistance. His body needed to be able to run without the machines. The feeding tube was working, and they were seeing benefits from that already.

"It will be a day of adjusting to these new things, resting and recovering," they told me.

Some days of rest for Nick were precisely what he needed, so it was great to see that happening. The doctors were back to the overall theme: with settings going down, we needed him to wake up. Every day Dr. Ng stressed it, ending our phone calls with: "He needs to wake up." I grew more and more anxious with each phone call. His eyes were opening now, but nothing was happening. We needed him to follow commands to show that he was making progress, that his brain was functioning. It was Good Shepherd Sunday, which made me feel invigorated. I hadn't know these Sundays existed before, but I now loved that they did. It was something to give us all hope.

I am Type A to my core. By ten a.m., I'd have already had my coffee, cleared my in-box, taught three classes, and returned home. Meanwhile, Nick would still be in bed.

When we first started dating, I noticed he would lie in bed and look at the ceiling for long stretches of time. It boggled my mind whenever I saw it.

What are you doing? I would think. *You are wasting so much time. You've been there for hours.*

Finally, one day I asked him. I had come back at noon from a full morning, and there he was—starring at the ceiling.

"What are you doing?" I exclaimed. "We have a matinee in two hours; you need to get up, shower, and go!"

I was not the first person to notice this.

His family called it "Nick time." I called it Fantasyland. Regardless, it was a time when Nick just zoned out, forgot about his responsibilities, and got lost in his thoughts. Every creative has a different process—I think Fantasyland was his.

He looked at me in all seriousness and said, "Babes, Fantasyland is important. Everyone needs Fantasyland."

He missed two matinees during *Bullets over Broadway* because of Fantasyland. I'm sure there were several creative things that came from Fantasyland, but he never shared them with me. So to me, these periods never made sense, they just seemed to make him late. His family later told me that "Nick time" had caused him to miss countless flights over the years.

Nick did things on his own time; he had his own internal clock.

I got off the phone with Dr. Ng and thought of Fantasyland for the first time. It dawned on me that instant—Nick was in Fantasyland right now. He doesn't want to wake up because he is in there thinking, learning. Nick loved to learn. He was the type of person who would stay up till four in the morning watching documentaries. This made me feel so much better.

I knew my husband; he would wake up when he was good and ready, not on the doctor's timetable . . . on his own. He was always late to the party.

I immediately called Lesley and told her.

"Mom, I think Nick is in Fantasyland! He's on 'Nick time' right now. That's why he isn't waking up yet. This is so like him to be late waking up, to be enjoying his thoughts right now. Fantasyland is important."

She laughed. "Amanda, you have a point there."

At times like this I felt like the whole journey we were on was like a jigsaw puzzle. I knew what the big picture was: I just had to turn over all the pieces and figure out how they all fit together. Nick couldn't talk to me, but as I searched for answers and help, I felt like I was finding signs he had left for me. "Live Your Life," Steph's sessions, Dr. John, the story of the Good Shepherd, and now Fantasyland . . . they were all pieces of the puzzle. I was slowly filling in the border, and I needed the big, middle pieces to come together.

I tried to rest as much as I could that week. Since I couldn't go into the hospital, I had no agenda but my business, three p.m. singing, and Elvis. Todd and Anna took Elvis on long car rides around Los Angeles so that I could have time to myself to work on everything. I had already begun telling Todd that he should leave San Francisco and move here—and Anna, she wasn't allowed to leave. They both needed to stay in Los Angeles forever. Of course, I was joking but also secretly hoping that Anna would fall in love with the city and decide to move here, and that Todd would relocate his family.

"I could quarantine with you two forever," I told them one day, and I meant it. They both laughed, agreeing with me. "I *know.* Why did we *ever* stop living together? This is the best! Who needs those other people we let into our lives," we joked.

"Boy," said Todd. "Maybe if Anna does move to California, I'll finally be in the circle."

"Biggie—what?" we said. "What circle?"

"Oh, there is a definite circle in this family, made up of you sisters, and I have always been on the outside of it."

"What?" we said again.

"I'll explain," he said, getting up from the table and grabbing the whiteboard and a marker from the fireplace mantel. He began drawing and narrating as he went.

"The secrecy of the sisters," he said, drawing three small circles and labeling them with our names.

"There are three separate secret holders: Anna and Amanda have their own secrets."

"True," we said.

"Anna and Traci have their own secrets."

"Definitely true," we confirmed.

He continued, "Alison only has secrets with Amanda, definitely not with Traci!"

"Huh, yeah," I said, realizing that was true.

"And Alison doesn't have any secrets with Anna."

"That is not true!" Anna interjected. "Alison and I definitely have our own secrets."

"Oh, wow, okay," said Todd.

"And then there's one thing I'm not certain about: an outer layer that contains things only the sisters know."

"That is true," I confirmed.

"And then," he said, frowning, "there's me," and he pointed to a dot he drew far away from everyone else. "On the out."

We burst out laughing.

He continued explaining as we laughed hysterically, realizing everything he was saying was, in fact, true. Among us sisters, we did have our own sets of secrets. Among all the sisters, there were group secrets. He complained things reached him only through Mom, or occasionally my older sister Alison. But Anna pointed out that any information that reaches anyone through my mom is not always accurate; it's usually exaggerated and rarely the real story.

He drew a squiggly line around the "sisters" circle, and labeled it "Mom" and called it "the distortion field."

"Now here's a question," he asked. "Why am I out here? What did I do? Seriously!"

He had his theories: because he was the oldest; because, for so long, he was the only one on the West Coast. But what it came down to was just that we had never really shared as many of our secrets with our brother as we did with each other.

"I'm just out here, on the out," he said.

He was joking, but of course, it was rooted in some truth. We hadn't been as close to Todd as we had with one another. But one of the silver linings of Nick's hospitalization and the quarantine was that that was really changing. The three of us were forming a bond that we could never have imagined, experiencing something as adult siblings that would never have happened in the real world.

"You're not far off, Biggie, but you can draw a new circle," Anna said. "The Amanda-Biggie-Anna circle. A new circle!"

"Yeah," I added. "I really do trust you both now, more than ever."

"Now that we're all out here, and we've gone through this together, things are gonna change! The circle will be reshaped," Anna said.

"Well," Todd sighed, picking up a chocolate chip cookie and taking a bite, "hopefully."

Todd is very close with his two boys, and when he packed up and drove to LA almost a month ago now, they didn't realize they'd be without their dad for so long. With Mother's Day coming up, and Anna fully trained in Elvis duties, and Nick in a more stable place, Todd was planning on going back to San Francisco. Until he did, we FaceTimed his kids every night as we ate dinner.

Anna and I would wake up every morning with bloated stomachs and faces and say to each other, "Do not let me eat dessert tonight."

We laughed so much that week, despite how scary things were. We were aware of how much we needed the release, needed to laugh. We were so thankful to have one another for that.

I was so thankful for the continued support from around the world. The daily three p.m. singing never got old to me. I couldn't believe how each day brought more people, more videos: swing dancing, jumping rope, full-family dance routines. One of my favorite videos came from a man in his nineties, living in a nursing home. He was standing up and holding on to his walker and dancing as best as he could, singing "Live Your Life." He had been following the story and rooting for Nick. Watching it would bring me to tears every time. Regardless if I could go into the hospital or not, I would go stand outside and sing, and pray, and talk to Nick.

I received an amazing video that week from the cast of *A Bronx Tale* re-creating "Live Your Life." Each time a video like this would come to me, I was blown away. It was so kind of the cast to come together like this. I knew it took hours of rehearsal to make it happen. Broadway is a family, and they take care of their own. All actors were all out of work, Broadway wouldn't be coming back for a long time, and they should have all been down. But there they were, singing and performing and rooting for Nick. The cast didn't just sing his song; they expanded on the music and vocals to make his song even better! I was in tears watching it.

I knew that when Nick woke up and realized what everyone was do-ing, what had happened while he was sleeping—he wouldn't know what to do. He wouldn't believe it. A video appeared from Linda Perry, one of the most famous music producers and songwriters in LA. Nick had met Linda with her business partner, Kerry Brown, only a couple weeks before he got sick. He was so excited to tell me that he got a meeting with Kerry to play him some music he had been working on. At the meeting, Linda walked in and briefly shook Nick's hand and listened to a song or two, giving him some great feedback. He came home that afternoon beaming.

"Babes, I got to play Linda Perry some of my music," he said. He couldn't wipe the smile off his face for hours. Now just weeks later, Linda was on her radio show covering his song. I was in disbelief, so I couldn't imagine how Nick would feel when he eventually woke up. She did an incredible cover of his song—slowed down, acoustic guitar—that hit you right in the gut. I had always told Nick that his music sounded so good on a female voice, and this proved my point. I realized how cool it was that his song could be interpreted in so many ways. Linda and Kerry said that's the mark of a great song. Later that day, I FaceTimed with Nick and told him the whole story, and played him Linda's cover. I wouldn't have been shocked if this was the thing that would have jolted him awake.

I'd often go to bed on a high after days like this, especially if, on top of it, the night ended with a great report from the hospital. But I was never safe from bad news the next morning. I never knew what to expect when I called the hospital just six hours later.

On May 5, Nick's oxygen levels had gone down overnight, which meant there were a lot of secretions in his lungs. This was a setback, and I was frustrated. We needed many stable days in a row. A day here or there wasn't good enough. For him to get better and wake up, we needed a steady week or two of no complications. *Where is our miracle, God?* I kept thinking.

My dad always has the best words of wisdom. He is the person we all call in a crisis. He always answers his phone, always keeps his cool, and always knows the right thing to say.

My dad offered some advice on the phone as I sat in silence that morning with my coffee. I told him that I kept praying for a miracle, and it wasn't happening. He said, "Amanda, you are getting your miracle every day. Nick is still here with us, so every day is a miracle. Every day your prayer is being answered."

Reality check. My dad was right, and I hadn't looked at it like that before.

Every day was a miracle. Nick could have died and left us on April 10—but he didn't.

It was May 5, and he was still here, still fighting. So I had to be there, too, still fighting.

I walked into Brown Bear to sneak up behind Todd and Elvis, watching Elmo.

"I didn't know that Elmo had a goldfish, did you, Elvito?" Todd asked him.

My heart melted. I have the best brother in the whole world.

Elvis looked back at him with his big, brown eyes, like, *Duh, Uncle Todd. Her name is Dorothy.*

The phone rang, the house stopped, and I answered. But this was one of those rare days when the hospital was calling with some good news. Nick's eyes were open, and there were very, very early signs that he may be waking up! One nurse thought she saw him tracking her. It was starting; he was waking up, and we couldn't contain our excitement. I instantly started crying because it was that one ounce of hope that I needed, that we all needed. It was so close to Mother's Day, and Anna had predicted over and over that he would wake up for me that day as my Mother's Day present. It was looking like that could happen now.

With Nick now on the trach, and possibly waking up soon, and Anna and me in a good flow, Todd decided to drive back to San Francisco. The night before he left we had a Cinco de Mayo party as a goodbye. Anna and I hated that he was leaving, but we understood. It felt like his leaving was the end of this little chapter of our story, this unique time in our lives as siblings. We had never had time with our brother like this, and we were both aware that we probably never would again. His leaving was breaking the little magic spell that was making everything work. It was a bit scary for me, and Anna, too. Todd knew things we didn't know—and without our brother around, we felt just a little less secure. He had taken care of me, and us, in so many ways. He was such a thoughtful and selfless person.

He told us as we hugged him with tears in our eyes that he was just a drive away and could come back whenever we needed him. We stood in a huddle for a long moment. No one wanted to let go, and as we slowly started to separate, Anna said, "Look, Biggie—it's the new circle!"

I told Todd he had arrived into trauma and was leaving with a triumph.

"Then my work here is done," he replied.

As he drove away, I hugged Anna so hard. We both were crying as he drove down Lookout Mountain, leaving the Canyon, and leaving us.

My army took his departure hard, too. I put Todd's driving away on Instagram, letting everyone know that he was going home, and I got thousands of replies.

People still tell me today, "I cried when Biggie left."

twelve

Despite all the sadness, fear, and uncertainty around us, Anna and I can't be in the same room and not make each other laugh. When Todd left, we felt it. We missed him so much. We missed his ten meals a day, his coffee runs, his funny notes, and his delicious dinners. Even today, when I think of the memories from that time, as awful as those days were, I find myself smiling, laughing, and missing those days, trapped together with nowhere to go and nothing to do but pray and dance and spend time with Todd, Anna, and Elvis.

In many ways, the virus came and took away everything we knew and relied on. Every distraction, every obligation, every social event—canceled. It left us with only relationships. The only things we could rely on were Zoom chats, phone calls, and the people with whom we were quarantining, if we were lucky enough to have them. I know, without a doubt, I could not have done this alone. I would've cracked after two weeks. But instead of falling apart, I spent the days strong and often even smiling. Due to Elvis, Todd, and Anna, I look back at these first forty days and miss them; in a weird way, I wish that I could relive them. Each day we were just trying to get through, waiting for it to be over. Now I wish they had never had to end.

In addition to what she was doing already, Anna had to take on the jobs Todd had been managing—and the role of cheerleader—because my morale dipped very low for the next week as the hospital refused, day after day, to let me in. Nick was showing early signs of waking up, and I wasn't allowed to be there to encourage him. I'm a personal trainer! Motivation is the name of my game. Instead, I FaceTimed him for an hour, twice a day. I tried to stay upbeat and positive, but these calls broke my heart. I went from playing with Elvis, to the depressing reality of Nick's hospital room, and it made me feel guilty that I was living a normal life at home, while he was alone in the hospital. I would completely break down after getting off the phone.

We made sure to exercise every day to release stress and offset all the dessert. "I don't know how I managed to do this, but I have definitely put on ten pounds in three weeks," Anna said. We laughed hysterically one night when she could not button her jeans that she had arrived with just a month before.

Elvis was changing so much every day; it simultaneously wowed me and pained me to watch. At this age, a baby goes to bed as one person and wakes up a completely different one. The day Todd was getting ready to leave, we realized that Elvis had finally learned how to tell us he was finished eating. We had been trying to teach him sign language for "all done" for months so he could communicate when he wasn't hungry anymore, but he wasn't getting it.

"All done," I would say to him, waving my hands each time before I took him out of his high chair.

It was Todd who noticed. He was trying to get him to eat, and Elvis was frantically waving his arms around.

"Hey! I think Elvis is doing 'all done'! I think he's finally learned it," he said.

And I observed and confirmed, "Oh my gosh, he *is* doing 'all done'!"

Elvis had finally learned it, and Nick wasn't here to see it.

He was crawling better and faster every day. He was growing more and more curious. You could entertain him for hours with just the buckles on his stroller or any kind of drawer. When his Stroller Buddies dropped him off, we got into the habit of taking him out of his stroller and letting him just play with it in the driveway because it kept him occupied for at least another forty-five minutes.

He was also becoming such a little lover, such a cuddle bug. I could hold him on the couch while I watched something mindless, and he would be content just to sit there cuddling on me until we both fell asleep.

Now that it was just Anna and me, we spent even more time together—she never left me to do an Instagram Live alone. We got into the habit of chatting together, still live, after singing. We talked about what was going on and anything and everything else that came to our mind. Sometimes they went on for an hour. It was fun; it felt as if we had other friends or were hosting our own talk show. We'd take questions from people on the Live and riff off each other. Our neighbor Molly started calling us a sitcom. "Can I be the strange neighbor who just pops in all the time?" she asked.

Meanwhile, Paris was back up and running. They had ended their quarantine on May 11. I was aware Anna could have gone home and started to resume the life she had begun there. I didn't want her to leave, but I felt like I had to tell her that she could if she wanted to. I knew I couldn't expect my entire family to stop their lives forever and live in Laurel Canyon with me. The doctor had told me more than once that this was a marathon, not a sprint. I knew we were in this for the long haul, and no one knew how long it would take for Nick to wake up, and then how long it would be before he could leave the hospital. Every day in the ICU meant a week in rehab. Nick had already been in the ICU for fifty days.

"Mandy," she said when I told her she could leave when she wanted to, "I'm not going anywhere. I will leave one day and go back to Paris for a little bit—I have all my stuff sitting there in the apartment, and I have to go get it at some point. But I'll only do that when someone else has come and been thoroughly trained in helping. The family has already talked about this."

It brought me to tears.

"We're not going to let you be alone at any point until Nick is home and healthy," she continued. "We're going to figure out shifts between me, Todd, Mom, and Dad, and whoever else can come out eventually. We may have to come and go, but there will always be someone here with you. There will always be a Kloots in the Canyon."

When you are living a trauma like this—it's easy just to focus on how much it is affecting you. But this made me realize how much something that happens to one person can affect an entire family. My parents had retired earlier that year and moved to New York. Their brand-new apartment was sitting there, waiting for them. Now I realized that instead of going back to it, they were planning to come to live here with me. They didn't know or like LA. They had wanted to be New Yorkers for years, and it had finally happened. I learned they were trying to get out of their lease, sell everything they had bought, and then spend most of the year helping me here.

Not being allowed to visit the hospital that week, I spent a lot of time on long phone calls with Dr. John, the private health-care team, and other doctors around the world trying to come up with ideas for treatments that could help Nick and ways to get me in the door. People were sending me suggestions every day that ranged in subject matter and seriousness: vitamin C, experimental stem cells, peptide injections, even rotating his bed so that it faced south. Most of the messages I got were repetitive, but I spent hours reading them, hoping someone had a new solution. I brought up anything to the doctors that I thought sounded hopeful.

It was exhausting, and it wore me down. One afternoon, I tried to lie down on the couch to take a nap, but Elvis wasn't tired.

"Why don't I take him on a walk?" Anna said. She scooped him up, walked out the door, and headed down the street.

When I woke up an hour later, she was just coming in the gate. She had Elvis on top of her shoulders and was holding his tiny hands in hers, bouncing him up and down, and he was smiling and laughing.

"Someone loves his auntie," I said to him when she walked in the door.

"I think I finally did it," Anna laughed. "I think he finally loves me!"

After that, Anna took Elvis on an hour's walk every day so that I could sleep or rest or do whatever I needed to do. She was determined to find new music for him to accept and add to his very selective play-list. She came back from a Canyon walk one day and said, "Mands—I found a new song that Elvis likes—'Rainbow' by Kacey Musgraves."

The lyrics to the song were the perfect anthem. It's about how some-times it feels like everything is going wrong and the world is crashing down on you, but you shouldn't be scared. You have to remember that after the rain will come a rainbow. *There's always been a rainbow hanging over your head.*

Elvis—who had seemingly the pickiest taste in music ever—liked this song and everything from the *Golden Hour* album.

To watch your siblings show your child so much love and care is a feeling that's hard to describe. Once you become a mom, you know you would do anything for your child. You would sacrifice anything, stop anything, do anything to make sure they were safe, protected, and loved. To know that while I was away, Elvis was with someone who loved him and cared for him the same way I would and that he was happy was a massive weight off my shoulders.

I was lying on the couch the night of May 9 after dinner, wearing an LED face mask to relax, and watching the first season of *Gilmore Girls*. The next morning was Mother's Day, and gifts had already been arriving for me all week. I was blown away by how many people were thinking of me on this holiday. It was my first official one since Elvis arrived, and we hadn't exactly celebrated the year before.

★   ★   ★

I woke up on Mother's Day 2019 with Elvis still in my belly. But I considered it my first Mother's Day. I was eight months pregnant, so I truly felt that I had earned my "mother" title already. I don't blame Nick for not knowing that I thought this was my first Mother's Day, but my feelings were hurt when I didn't wake up to a celebration.

My siblings and I grew up "over-celebrating" everything in life and always looking for ways to make a celebration out of otherwise ordinary things. Every holiday called for the good china and crystal, both sets of grandparents, a big family dinner, and at least three desserts to feed us all. We went out as a family to celebrate every recital, performance, band show, or game. Our birthdays, growing up, were the biggest ordeal. As the birthday boy or girl slept, the rest of the family decorated his or her bedroom with handmade posters, signs, and balloons. The decorations often extended into the kitchen or living room of the house, too. There would be a mountain of presents, an enormous cake, and a thick stack of cards that, as they were opened, went on display around the kitchen and stayed there for a few weeks. We were always like this as a family, and it's something we never grew out of. Even as adults, we love cards, banners, and confetti, and always decorate the house for one another on special days. I had been expecting something.

I woke up and took our two dogs on a walk to give Nick a chance to "set up" the surprise I imagined he was planning, but I came back home to find him still in bed.

We had my niece's baptism that morning, so we quickly got ready for church. It was a monsoon outside. As we walked, our umbrella flipped inside out because it was so windy and cold. I sat through the service, crying my eyes out. I went through tissue after tissue and could not stop. It was emotional seeing my niece being baptized, and I was also emotional feeling as if Nick didn't think it was important to celebrate me. I was having a Mother's Day meltdown. Nick had no idea that my tears had anything to do with him.

After church and brunch, I thought he still had some time to redeem himself. Maybe he was taking me out for dinner? Maybe there was a card at home?

"What should we do for dinner?" I finally asked around five.

"I don't know, babes, you feeling pizza?" he asked.

I burst into tears again, finally confessed to him that I was sad that he hadn't recognized this day for me. It was a classic *Men Are from Mars* moment; he looked so shocked and confused. We didn't have a baby yet.

He confessed to me, sheepishly, that he didn't see it that way; he didn't think that this *was* my first Mother's Day.

When you have spent eight months growing, naming, and bonding with the child inside you—you beg to differ. But we agreed to disagree. I knew he hadn't meant to hurt my feelings and didn't really think that my carrying our child was unimportant. Elvis was the most important thing to both of us now. Nick was equal parts excited and terrified about becoming a dad because he had been unemployed for almost a year. He was desperate for work, auditioning for everything and anything so that we could raise Elvis in a good neighborhood, with a good school, and never have to worry about providing for him. Nick and I saw eye to eye on most things about raising our family. But that night, I realized, I was going to have to give him a crash course in celebrations.

Mother's Day ended with a pizza delivery and Netflix on the couch.

You can make up for it next year, I thought as we sat there.

I feel guilty for thinking that now.

This year, I knew the celebration wouldn't be normal either. There was nothing to do and nowhere to go. Our neighbor Jono had continued the Sunday series he'd started weeks earlier, so we planned to go to that. I usually love celebrating, but everything just felt off.

When I woke up the next morning, the kitchen and living room were entirely decorated. The whiteboard was front and center and had been repurposed into a poster that read, "Happy Mother's Day, Mands!" Anna had taken all the presents that had come and put them into a massive pile on the kitchen table. There was a giant, heart-shaped, Happy Mother's Day balloon, and she had used colored construction paper to make paper hearts that she taped all over the walls that said things like, YOU ARE AN INSPIRATION, YOU ARE STRONG, YOU ARE AMAZING. When she got up, she made me banana pancakes, and we called the hospital to FaceTime with Nick.

He had been on a great streak. The doctors were now certain his tracking and movement were wake-up signs, and we were all thrilled. What he needed to happen most was happening! When the nurse connected us, Nick's eyes were wide open, wider than they had been before.

"Honey, it's Amanda. It's so lovely to see your eyes! Can you hear me, Nick?"

He was looking right at me.

"Blink if you can hear me, Nick."

As if in slow motion, Nick's eyelids shut and reopened. He was so weak that just to perform that tiny motion took him thirty seconds. But he did it.

"He's moving, he's responding, Mands," Anna shouted. "Way to go, brother!"

I grabbed Elvis to show him to Nick.

"Nick, this is Elvis, your son. Look up if you know who Elvis is," I said.

Again, in slow motion, he looked up.

I was overjoyed. We were cheering, smiling, and in disbelief. He was communicating with us.

I asked the nurse who was with him, "Are you seeing this? Is he awake?"

She responded, "I am seeing it! He is definitely responding. I need to update the doctors, and they'll assess his mental status to be sure, but I think he is definitely aware. I think he's woken up."

We stayed on FaceTime singing, talking, and asking him questions, and his eyes were moving the entire time. But eventually, the eye movements took so much out of him that his eyelids got heavy again, and he drifted off to sleep. This was more action than he had seen in forty days! We couldn't totally confirm anything yet, but it felt like there was no way this meant something else. I didn't want to celebrate too soon, but when I hung up, I was overjoyed. It was the only gift I needed.

My table of gifts was like Christmas morning. I had received things from everyone I knew and people I didn't know. My cousins and family all went in and bought me a beautiful set of wind chimes for the new house. There were flower deliveries and clothes and custom #wakeupnick masks. Anna, of course, wanted to get me a gift but didn't know what to do. She couldn't go out and go shopping, and since she was witnessing all the daily deliveries—she knew I didn't actually need a thing. A few days before, she had asked me what I wanted to have for dinner and offered to cook or order whatever I wanted. But she had been trying to come up with ideas of what to give me, too, and nothing made sense.

She had seen me writing Elvis one of his letters one night at the kitchen table. After the initial one in early April, I wrote one every week so he'd have his own "Dear Elvis" time capsule. On Mother's Day, she explained there was nothing she could think of to buy me, but she had written her own "Dear Elvis" letter about what I was like as a mom.

"I wanted you to know and him to know what an amazing mom you are. Everything I see you doing—you may not realize—is so extraordinary. You're the best mom to him, Mandy, so I wrote this so you would see it, in case you ever doubt it."

Dear Elvis,

It's your mom's first Mother's Day, and to use the same words that your dad did in her birthday card—it is not the kind she wanted or deserves. But she woke up this morning as she always does—with a full heart and a smile.

You're eleven months old today. You don't know or understand what is going on in the world right now or what has happened to your family, and for that, I am so grateful. You don't feel the fear, or uncertainty, or understand the drastic change that has occurred in our daily lives—especially you and your mom's. That is due to your age, but it is also due to her. Her spirit that never wavers, her smile that never fades, and her faith that never fails. She uses it all to shield you from the bad—so that you only feel goodness, and joy, and love every day.

She has been writing you letters so that one day you will be able to look back and know what happened when you were just a little, baby boy, our "petit." You will be able to read about how things changed so quickly, how our world stopped, and how slowly our Earth healed from it. You will understand why we always linger a second longer now when we hug and why we never miss a birthday party, a wedding, or a holiday. You will know why your mom and Uncle Todd and I are bonded in the most unbreakable way now.

But there are some things she's not telling you in her letters, things she won't come out and say herself, and so I'm writing you this one so that you will know. Elvis, you don't have a regular mom. You have a super mom.

Right now, you get into everything. You destroy the perfectly clean house in a matter of seconds. You open every cabinet you shouldn't touch and play with everything but your toys. You try to take down paintings, topple tables, and splash in the toilet. Everything you pick up, try to put right into your mouth—from dirty shoes to rocks, to the lemons that fall from the tree in the backyard. She never yells. She's never frustrated. She never, ever shouts. She looks at you with eyes that outpour admiration and laughs as you get into mischief. She lures you away from trouble with hugs, and cuddles, and games. Elvis, she is crazy about you.

And you're crazy about her, too. You really don't let her go out of your sight without instant tears. You want her to hold you ALL the time. You wrap your tiny arms around her neck and hold on tight to the collar of her shirt. She can't really shower, or make a phone call, or even pour a cup of coffee without you in her arms. She does not get a minute for herself. Not one. But she never complains, not even for a second. She holds you close and kisses you one thousand times each hour, and tells you over, and over, and over again, "I LOVE YOU SO MUCH."

And if she does have to put you down because the doctors are calling and something has happened to your dad, she comes to scoop you back up the second that she can. She might have red eyes and freshly-wiped-away tears, but she sees you and breaks into a wide smile, and so do you. Then you desperately do your strange one-legged scoot across the floor toward her at an alarmingly fast pace.

"Hey," she says, picking you up, "I MISSED YOU!"

Elvis, she is a warrior.

What has happened to your dad is sometimes impossible to

believe. So much, so quickly—it feels to us like it can't be real. Your mom has dealt with more fear, and pain, and stress in the last six weeks than most people could ever endure in a lifetime. She was doing it all alone, and rather than become consumed by the sad reality of emptiness, the way so many people would have, she created a virtual army. She asked people all over the world to pray, and sing, and believe so that you two would not be here alone in this fight.

She has you talk to your dad every day. You smile at him through FaceTime. You coo, and squeak, and giggle, and she talks for you because you don't have the words yet.

"I LOVE YOU, DADA," she says into the phone.

"I MISS YOU, DADA, WAKE UP!"

You dance, and cheer, and pray for your dad every single day. She makes sure that you do.

Elvis, she's an inspiration.

When you nap or sleep, she should too—but instead, she works. She gives a free workout to the world; she researches rehab centers and prosthetics and talks to COVID survivors.

When you're awake, she plays with you on the floor, she teaches you how to do sit-ups, she chases you around the house on all fours saying "I'm gonna get you," as you squeal. She dances with you and plays peek-a-boo, which makes you laugh so hard, and right now, I promise it's the best sound in the world. She will sing "The Wheels on the Bus" for an hour straight if that's what it takes to keep you happy. And while I want to gouge my ears out after five minutes of it, she is still smiling with every single verse. And so are you. She never stops.

Elvis, she is one-of-a-kind.

I have never seen someone give someone else the kind of pure and selfless love that your mom gives you. You hit the

jackpot, kid, getting her for a mom. I know, because I hit the jackpot, too, when I got her for a sister.

I was in tears two paragraphs in. I hadn't realized all of this, all that
we were going through and doing, but she captured it in such a moving way. I was getting through each day the only way I knew how, and
reading Anna's letter was the first time I heard what the days were like
looking in. It was the perfect gift.

At five p.m., we headed down to the corner to participate in the
Mother's Day sing-along that Jono had organized. He was always looking for ways to bring the community together and help people through
song. Jono had a big, hand-painted LIVE YOUR LIFE banner across his
gate, which he kept up until the very end. There were maybe just ten of
us there that first evening, the original founding members of the Laurel
Canyon Community Choir. He had an amp and microphone set up, and
Bill was there, too, on his keyboard.

Jono welcomed everyone and announced that we were going to sing
three songs: "Sing a Song" by the Carpenters, "You've Got a Friend" by
Carole King, and "Live Your Life" by Nick Cordero.

We all stood in the street on the warm, spring night as the sun was
setting. We stood far away from each other, wearing our masks, but we
felt connected as we began to sing. "Sing of good things not bad, sing
of happy not sad . . ."

It was a double-edged sword attending music nights. On the one
hand, it was exactly what Nick would have wanted me to do, wanted us
to do. He would have been there with bells on and a guitar in his hands
if he could have. But being part of these Canyon music nights gutted me
for the exact same reason. He would have loved them so much, but he
couldn't see them or participate in them. Anna and I stood in the street
that evening, arms around each other, and swayed back and forth as we
sang "You've Got a Friend."

Later, at home, Anna made dinner. I had decided my dream meal was a cheese quesadilla, wine, and the confetti cake that my best friend had sent. I've never been a fancy eater, and a simple cheesy quesadilla sounded perfect. I scooped big blobs of sour cream onto the top, and Anna put out some of the chips and salsa we had left over from our Cinco de Mayo party.

It wasn't fancy, it wasn't elaborate, but it was perfect. Then we devoured the rest of the amazing banana bread that my friend Lauren's mom had made for us earlier in the week.

Nick had been responsive. He had opened his eyes and knew that I was there. Last year, I had thought he better do something big this year—and by waking up on Mother's Day, he had gone above and beyond.

The next morning when I called the hospital, I asked for Dr. Ng.

"Dr. Ng," I asked, "he was tracking, and blinking on command, and looking right at me yesterday! Even his jaw moved! There were times I felt like he was trying to say something, but then realized he can't!"

"It's just going to take a bit of time, but he's going in the right direction. He's getting more and more stable; we are making slow and steady improvements."

I was afraid even to ask the question, but I had to.

"Then, Doctor," I said, "would you say that . . . You know our theme has been, 'We gotta wake him up!' Can we say that he's woken up? Is he awake?"

"I think he's up. He's following commands. He's definitely up," he said. "It's a process; if he wasn't so profoundly weak, he'd be doing more. It's just a lot of fallout from how much he's gone through. He could certainly be more awake than this, but he'll continue to improve! He's no longer in a coma."

We cheered, hugged, and cried through breakfast. I grabbed Elvis and hugged him, telling him, "Dada is awake!"

Then I told everyone. Family, friends, our neighbors! I felt like running through the streets, screaming it. I got on Instagram and shared it in a story while holding Elvis in the frame. It was soon picked up by the news, and then the whole world knew.

My friends here in the Canyon—our little quaranteam—were all overjoyed.

"We've got to pop champagne!" Anna said.

We invited the team to come over for a socially distanced celebratory toast in the driveway that night. The doctors had been saying "He needs to wake up!" And now he was up. It was the huge hurdle we finally leaped over, and it felt like now we were on the home stretch of this marathon.

Anna had been saying all along, "This is game seven," referring to the year the Cleveland Cavaliers won the NBA finals, against all the odds. Everyone counted them out, but in the end, they won the way no one else has ever won in history, and that made it all the more monumental. Today, we felt like we had just won the NBA finals. We had all been working so hard as a team, and this was a real moment of victory. It was the only one we got.

I got to FaceTime with Nick a few hours later, after they were done with another bronch. He was more responsive than ever. Moving his eyes around, and up and down, to answer the questions we were asking him. I was communicating again with my husband for the first time in over a month.

"I'm going to get back in there, honey, don't you worry," I told him as we hung up. "They kicked me out, but they're not going to keep me out! I can't wait to see you, sweetheart; I love you!"

Now that Nick was awake, I was fixated on getting into the hospital, and each day they wouldn't let me in enraged me. I grew more frustrated on every call with the nurses, trying to get to the bottom of exactly whom I had to convince and what I had to do to convince them.

Dr. John and I would talk multiple times a day. He was my sounding board before I suggested things to Dr. Ng, and spent hours each day on the phone with doctors all over the world, looking for solutions.

I was learning how a hospital is a business, for better or worse. There are groups and hierarchies and boards. So many boards. I might seem naive, but I had no idea that this was how hospitals were assembled. Daily, people all over the country were working on my behalf, begging, pleading, and bartering with these boards to try to get me into the hospital. With the guidance of Dr. John and Dr. Ng and the work of countless others, I felt very grateful for all the help from people who were doing what they could to get me inside to see him. I kept praying every day that it would work.

Through all the persistence, I don't know what finally did it, but I received a phone call from Debra, which was then confirmed by Dr. Ng, that the doctors had decided it would be a good idea for us all to do a weekly status meeting at the hospital. This would ensure I got to see Nick once a week and would have time to review with the doctors Nick's progress and the plans for the week. They decided I should come in every Monday.

I called Dr. John right away and asked if I could conference him in on these meetings. John was so great at listening to what the doctors said and then explaining it all to me afterward. He also asked the doctors questions during the meetings that I didn't even know to ask. I had to share the good news and thank him! It was definitely his work that got me in there.

"Amanda," he said. "Bring treats when you go."

"Huh?" I said.

"Do you bake?" he asked. "Arrive with cookies or something every week. Homemade is better. It shows you really care."

I went into an excited anxiety attack because I was so nervous. I would do whatever it took. But I was also shocked that *baking* is what was finally going to get me into the door at Cedars? I didn't have time to bake anything. I didn't have any ingredients at the house, and I had Elvis attached to my leg. John said baked is better than bought, so I ran to the Canyon Country Store to grab supplies.

I never bake and don't have any "go-to" recipes for treats. I had only a few hours until I had to leave and didn't have time to make anything too elaborate. But I had once made cake balls with a friend, so it came to my mind to do something like that. I didn't have time to bake a cake, but I found a recipe that used Oreos and thought, *Perfect!*

Back at Brown Bear, Anna had just gotten home from her run, and I explained everything as I started tearing apart the package of Oreos and dumping them on a cutting board, Oreo crumbs scattering across the countertop. I got out the huge chef's knife and started trying to chop up the cookies; the recipe called for crushed Oreos, but I didn't know how to crush them. Bits of Oreos were flying everywhere as I frantically hacked at them and told Anna, "I gotta make these as soon as I can, and then take them to the hospital, and they will let me in! Can you just watch Elvis while I do this?"

She was looking at me like a deer in headlights; wondering how to prevent the quickly approaching disaster.

"Mandy, this is excellent news. I am so happy for you. Are you sure about this recipe, though? Oreo truffles are kind of complicated and messy to make with the crushing, and then you need to use a double boiler to melt the chocolate, and dip them, and cool them, and keep them refrigerated . . . Did you buy paraffin wax?"

"Paraffin what?" I asked

"Oh boy," she said. "Why don't I help you, and we can use the Oreos but make something else?"

She was being reasonable, but I was crazed. I had started, and I was determined to finish.

"No, I can do this," I said, still chopping like a madwoman. "I want to make these. They are easy to eat and share. A nurse can just walk by, pick one up, pop it in, and go. I've done this once before. It's not hard." I was struggling with the knife as I said it. "I just need to crush these damn Oreos!"

Anna continued to try to reason with me, saying we had everything to whip up some Oreo brownies instead, which would be easy, would take only one pan, and would be ready in thirty minutes flat. But her fighting me on this was just making me mad, and I got more and more stubborn about doing this recipe and making them myself.

"Please, Amanda," she finally begged. "This is a bad idea. You're going to make a huge mess, and they are not going to work out in the end. Let me do this for you."

I pulled the lid off of the blender and started scooping handfuls of the Oreos into it to try to crush them that way. I replaced the top and hit start, but it just made a terrible, grinding noise.

I screamed. All my frustration at the hospital was finally coming out physically. I was taking it out on the Oreos. I yanked the lid of the blender off, dumped the contents back onto the board, and resumed frantically chopping.

"Okay, that's it," Anna said sternly.

She came over, took the knife away from me, and said, "You're going to hurt yourself and or destroy this kitchen. I'm taking over, and I'm making Oreo brownies. You are banned from the cabin. Go walk around outside. Take Elvis. You can come back in thirty minutes. I mean it. Out!"

When I came back in thirty minutes, the kitchen was magically spotless, Kacey Musgraves was playing softly, and the house smelled like warm chocolate.

Bibbidi-Bobbidi-Boo!

Not long after, I left for the hospital to see Nick, with two dozen perfect Oreo brownies in the passenger seat next to me.

thirteen

Nick had been asleep for forty days. I knew this, but my sister Traci was the first to point out to me the biblical significance of that length of time.

When I looked it up online, I found, "The number forty is particularly connected to the fulfillment of God's plans, and not all of them positive. It is often associated with the theme of testing, trials, and judgment."

Countless examples came right back to me from Bible study.

- The rains fell on Noah's ark for forty days and nights (Genesis 7:4).
- Moses was with God on the mountain, forty days and nights, without eating bread or water (Exodus 24:18, 34:28).
- David reigned over Israel for forty years (2 Samuel 5:4, 1 Kings 2:11).
- Egypt to be laid desolate for forty years (Ezekiel 29:11–12).
- Jesus fasted forty days and nights (Matthew 4:2).
- Jesus was tempted forty days (Luke 4:2, Mark 1:13).
- Jesus remained on Earth forty days after the resurrection (Acts 1:3).

I wasn't sure what it all meant, but by this point, I was convinced that God was talking to Nick. There were too many parallels to simply ignore them.

I sat in the same cold, concrete room we had used the last time the doctors had called me in. It was Dr. Ng, Dr. Welch, Dr. Williams, Nick's nurse for that day, and Debra.

I finally had everyone in one place, and I could ask questions and get all the opinions at the same time. Their thoughts on Nick's health were rarely the same, but at least I could hear them all talk together here—rather than the way things had been going.

The doctors were concerned. Nick had woken up but had not shown any improvement. He was so profoundly weak he couldn't do anything and was still on assistance from the vent. They had tried to lower his PEEP (positive end-expiratory pressure) a few times that week but had to raise it right back up each time. Nick had been in a cycle for a while of making small improvements, but then something bad would happen—an infection, septic shock, a sudden dip in blood pressure—that would undo all the progress. They could get him back to stable, but never back to the level he had been at previously. Each time something happened to him, his overall health dipped considerably, and he never fully recovered. He was plateauing. We needed a plan to start seeing results.

Dr. John was there with me on speakerphone, armed and ready with a list of questions.

"What about high-dose steroids?" he started.

"There's little to no evidence that would work," the doctors said.

"And this is probably a crazy idea, but is a lung transplant something you're considering?" he asked.

"No, that wouldn't be something that we are considering at this time," they replied.

A lung transplant? I thought. *Oh my God, is that actually something that might happen?*

The thought of that sounded drastic, desperate, and scary. We couldn't be at that point—or get to it—could we?

I did a lot of listening in this meeting. I was learning. Learning about Nick, learning who these people were, learning what questions I could ask. It was so nice to have Dr. John on this call because I even learned from him. He was not afraid to ask questions, even if they seemed ridiculous. What did he have to lose?

The plan at the end of the meeting was to stay on course. We would keep moving forward at an aggressive pace. Nick was forty-one years old, *forty-one*. He had a life, a baby to live for. We would keep going.

After the meeting was over, I got to visit Nick. I ran into the room and by his side to see what kind of reactions I could get out of him now that he was awake. His eyes were open and were looking around—but not necessarily connected to anything. I wasn't sure he knew I was there. He had been so alert on the phone, so awake.

I struggled to get him to focus and look at something. At times I felt like he was, but then, minutes later he'd be gone, off into space. It was frustrating for me to have only this short time with him. He was tired and not as aware as when I'd FaceTimed with him. If I could be here all the time, I could catch him at his best. With this system, it was the luck of the draw. When my time was up, I had to leave the hospital, leave him there alone. It pained me every single time, walking out that door, knowing I was leaving him with no one.

When I got home that evening, I googled and researched lung transplants. I didn't like what I saw. It was a dangerous and lengthy surgery with a long donor list, and one's life span after surgery is ten years, at best. It was too terrifying to keep reading. Besides, the doctors today made it seem like we would never get to the point of a transplant. I closed my computer and turned on the TV instead.

Anna had noticed a shift in my mindset, and she alerted the family that I was feeling down, that they should try to be upbeat and positive when they called. Finally she took it upon herself to help me find a positive distraction.

When lockdown first began, Anna and I talked on FaceTime every night before she came here. I remembered that one day she said that she wasn't going to let this time pass and have nothing to show for it. She needed to create something, to do something productive.

"Hey, sister," I said one day, watching her go through emails over coffee.

"What if we started our business? We're together, in the same place for a while, with nothing to do! We're both out of work! Why not try it now?"

We'd had an idea back in January for a T-shirt company that we wanted to call Hooray For.

The idea came to us while watching Nick perform in *Rock of Ages* at the Bourbon Room. The narrator appeared onstage wearing a HOORAY FOR BOOBIES T-shirt. I poked Anna, pointed at the shirt, and said with a laugh, "I want that shirt!"

"I want 'Hooray for Cake,'" Anna replied. "And glitter, and Paris, and sisters, and . . . oh my God, this is a great idea!"

We spent the entire night writing down a list of all the things we wanted to say hooray for. Family, love, miracles, sunshine, dogs, cats, frosting, pizza . . . the list went on forever. HOORAY FOR EVERYTHING!

We started the research and planned to do it, but life got in the way of our getting Hooray For up and running. Anna moved to France, and I was already running a business and was a new mom. We knew it was a great idea, but we didn't have time to start it. But why not now? Now, more than ever, the world needed some happiness. The world needed to be reminded there were still good things out there, little blessings worth celebrating: sisters, love, family, sunshine, wine, friends! It was time to start Hooray For. We needed jobs, and the world needed some happiness.

We woke up every day to trauma and tragedy—but rather than focusing on the bad, we were choosing to count our blessings. When things got hard, we just reminded ourselves that we were lucky to be healthy and alive.

We can start with 'Hooray for Life'!" I said.

Anna loved it. "Sister, let's do it!" she agreed.

"But we need to give back," she added. "We need to donate some of the proceeds to help COVID research."

At that time, so many beautiful things were being done for us. People were dropping off meals and sending gifts, and flowers, and care packages. They took Elvis on walks, played us live music, and delivered fresh veggies from their gardens. We also knew what the Cedars-Sinai team was sacrificing to care for COVID patients because we saw it every day.

We knew how many people were suffering, and this was a chance to do something to help, to give back because so much was being given to us. We started making calls and ordering samples and researching organizations to donate to. Hooray For was born, and starting this business was something exciting, something that I really needed just then.

Not long after, I got to visit Nick in the hospital because the doctors had set up another family meeting with me. The ICU rotates doctors every two weeks, and there was a new doctor I was going to meet. I had not been allowed to see Nick for over a week, so I was anxious to get there.

However, a pit formed in my stomach when I received the morning call from the hospital. I was supposed to go in at three p.m., but they wanted to move it up.

"The doctors want you to come in earlier—Nick had a bad morning. Is one p.m. okay? Can you get here? They want to have a meeting."

Something didn't feel right. When I got to the car, I was frozen. I needed to start driving to the hospital, or I'd be late, but I couldn't move. I decided I needed to hear "Carry On" by Fun, my song to encourage me to start the car and get moving. I knew that the doctors were not going to give me good news. I needed to get over there, but I couldn't bring myself to step on the gas.

It is crazy how hearing a song can jolt you right back to another time and place in your life. One of the Broadway shows I performed in, *Follies*, had been doing a stint in Los Angeles at the Ahmanson Theatre. It was a dream gig because the show had closed on Broadway, and then a couple months later, we got a call saying they wanted to take the show to LA for a few months. I couldn't wait to come back to LA to perform with this show. I decided to live with my three closest friends in the cast during the stay in a little apartment behind The Grove at Park La Brea. Every day I would go for a long walk through the pretty neighborhoods for my exercise, listening to the new album by the band Fun. I would blast it in my ears, sing along, and power walk through the streets of LA. One of the songs on the album was titled "Carry On," and about three quarters of the way into it, the beat becomes triumphant and makes you feel like you can pull through anything. It was by far my favorite song on the album. This album, that song in particular, always brings me right back to living in LA and going on morning walks, imagining I can get through anything, knowing I can carry on.

When I got to the hospital, I met the ICU doctor—a young woman who had been with Nick before but I had never met. It was hard being introduced to new doctors on the regular at a time when I just craved some kind of consistency. Dr. Ng, Dr. John, and Debra were also in attendance. We were in our usual small conference room, down a hall from Nick's room. I barely walked through the doors before Debra showed me to the meeting space.

We all sat around the table wearing our masks. As always, the room felt airless.

"Nick is now in a state of severe acidosis. He is unable to release

CO_2 from his lungs, and that has caused his pH levels to be so dangerously low that his body can't function correctly. If your body can't recover from this state, you can experience kidney failure, respiratory failure, and you're likely to have a stroke." Nick could not have survived any of that.

"All his settings are at the maximum. He has copious amounts of phlegm in his lungs. It is bad, very bad. His infection isn't getting any better, despite his being on every antibiotic. There isn't another antibiotic that he could be on, and what he's on isn't helping. He is on a lot of blood pressure medications, but his blood pressure keeps dropping despite that. The numbers are very low. If they continue going lower, there's nothing we can do."

I kept it together. I didn't cry. I didn't overreact. I listened and asked all the questions that I could think of. John asked questions, as well. It was nice to have someone advocating on my behalf, asking questions I didn't know to ask, couldn't ask.

"Where is Nick's family?" one of the ICU doctors asked.

"Canada," I answered.

"Can they get here?" he said.

"What?"

He continued, "If they can get here, they should come. Now. Is there anyone you want here with you today?"

I couldn't even react because I didn't understand what they were getting at.

"Aren't you living with your sister?" the doctor asked. "We can let her in to be with you today if you want."

The confusion must have been visible on my face.

Debra chimed in, "You might need some support today, and we think we could get her cleared."

Is he not going to make it? I thought. *Are they saying he is going to die today?*

"Amanda," they said. They sounded a thousand miles away.

"Call your sister. Tell her to come. Tell Nick's family, too. We don't expect him to make it through the day."

I left the boardroom in a daze and started to walk to Nick's room, finally letting the tears fall as I called Nick's mother.

"Mom," I said, "they're saying Nick isn't going to make it and that you should get here if you can."

I didn't believe the words as I was saying them. This was coming out of left field for me, so I couldn't imagine how thrown off she would be. Lesley was stunned. She was barely responding to me, and I understood why. This had come out of nowhere. We had talked weeks ago about her coming, but we all agreed that it made more sense for her to come when she could stay, like when Nick was in rehab. Lesley was in Canada and did not think for one second that Nick wouldn't recover. I could tell she was trying to figure out how she could get there, who could come with her, whether she could get across the border, and if she could get here in time . . .

"Are you sure?" she asked. Over and over again she asked the same thing.

"That's what they're telling me, Mom. They're telling me that you need to get here."

She hung up to call Nick's brother and sister, Matt and Amanda, and tell them what I had just told her. Together the three of them decided to book the next flight so they could fly together and try to get here in time to say goodbye.

I texted Anna and told her I needed her at the hospital. She was in my bedroom, lying in the dark, with Elvis asleep on her chest. The whole world changed as she read my text. No one was prepared for this; it didn't make any sense. But she knew not to question me or ask for clarification. She just had to figure out how to get to the hospital. Our Canyon quaranteam came to the rescue: Rachel, Zach, and Florence appeared right away. Rachel put Elvis in his stroller for a walk while Molly pulled up in her car to drive Anna to Cedars-Sinai. Anna called Todd on the way to the hospital, and ten minutes later, he was packing his bag to return to Laurel Canyon.

I walked into Nick's room, all the doctors and nurses behind me. Nick looked bad. He was gray, not a trace of color in his face. I had never watched someone die, but this certainly looked a lot like I imagined it. I was with Nick, holding his hand and rubbing his head, tears pouring down my face. The instant I saw him, I understood what the doctors were saying. Once I was in the room, it all became even more real. The small anteroom started filling up with what seemed like all the sixth-floor nurses and doctors. It wasn't just Nick's team; everyone was coming by, looking at Nick, and me, and Nick's machines. The numbers, which I knew all too well by now, were bad—very, very bad. I got scared.

Debra walked into the room, and I told her that I had called Anna to be with me. "She can come in, right?" I asked.

Debra said she would make sure Anna was on the list.

The new ICU doctor came into the room and sat down beside me.

"Do you have any questions?" she asked.

"If he goes soon, how will it happen?" I asked. "I need to be prepared."

I didn't know what to expect. She put her arm around me and described how we would see the numbers continue to drop, especially the blood pressure. Then the oxygen saturation rate would get low. It's supposed to stay as close to 100 as possible; right now, it was in the 80s, but it had dropped even lower that morning.

"He will code," she said. "Do you want us to try to resuscitate him if that happens?"

I was hearing things in slow motion, so I was not fully understanding. Dr. Ng, who was also in the room, repeated the question.

I said, "Will it hurt him to do that? I don't want to put him through any more than he already has been through."

They told me it would be an added stress on his body, and it most likely would not save his life.

"Then no," I said. "I can't put him through any more."

So I sat there with a room full of nurses and doctors who had all been rooting for Nick. I was crying so hard, snot was running down my face and my mask was completely ruined.

The doctors and nurses were all looking at me like we didn't have much time. I didn't know what to do. In many ways, I had been prepared for this for a while, but I wasn't ready for today to be the day. There had been no warning signs. He had just woken up a week ago. I started making phone calls to immediate family and friends to FaceTime with him to say their goodbyes. They were put on the spot and improvised their goodbyes to Nick. Nick was unresponsive, back in his sleep state, his eyes almost closed. Tears rolled down my face as I listened to family and friends saying their goodbyes.

"When will his family arrive—what was the soonest flight they could get on?" the other ICU doctor asked me when he came in the room.

"Lesley and his sister and brother are on the next flight. They think they'll be here around noon tomorrow," I responded.

"We can do our best to keep him alive until they arrive, if you want," he said, "or we can move him into comfort care."

"Comfort care? What is that?" I asked.

He explained it meant that they would slowly start taking him off the machines, allowing his body to naturally drift off. At the same time, they would medicate him so that he wouldn't feel any pain.

"No," I said. "I'm not doing that. Please let's keep him alive until they arrive; Lesley needs to see her son."

Everyone finally left me alone in Nick's room, but his anteroom remained full. I sat by his side, gripping his hand, praying for his life. All the doctors and nurses on the other side of the glass doors were staring at the machines, noting his blood pressure, oxygen saturation rate, and heart rate. I understood the numbers now. Blood pressure needs to stay above 65. Oxygen saturation rate needs to be 90 to 100, with 100 being the best. The heart rate must remain above 60. Nick's blood pressure was dropping into the low 40s, and his saturation rate was sinking into the 50s. As I looked at the numbers, I believed what they were telling me: that he wouldn't make it through the night. Every time the numbers dropped, I'd squeezed his hand harder and tell him, "Nope. Come on, Nick. Not today, let's go, baby!"

I would rejoice if one of the numbers went up, even a notch.

Finally, those in the anteroom drifted away, and I had Nick to myself.

"Hi, honey. Honey, I love you. I love you so much. I don't know why this is happening to you. Why is this happening to you?"

I held him as much as I could, trying not to disturb all the wires and tubes.

"Babe, you have fought so hard. Thank you so much for fighting for me, for us. I know you're probably so tired, I cannot imagine. If you can still fight, please, please do. Please fight, honey. I need you. Elvis needs you. He needs his dad. I don't know what I'll do without you. Can you still fight for us, honey?"

More tears, more tissues.

"If you can't, though, if you can't, I understand. I want you to know that I will make sure Elvis knows you. He will learn about his dad, how amazing you are! I promise you that I will do everything, *everything* I can for that little boy. He looks just like you, babes. Oh my God, he is the cutest little guy. I promise you to be the best mom I can possibly be, okay? I'm going to pray with you, honey. You always liked—or you said you did, at least—that you liked when I prayed, so let's pray."

Dear God, thank you for my husband. Thank you for this man. God, please don't take him from me. Please save him, Lord. Send your angels down right now, have mercy on him, Lord. Please. Please don't take him. I believe in miracles, and you are the miracle giver. You and only you have the power to grant Nick a miracle. Give him a miracle. I still have faith, it may be as small as a mustard seed, but I have it.

I was holding Nick's hand, rubbing his arm, his head, his hair as I prayed.

But God, if you need him . . . I will never understand it. I will try to, I will try my best to, it will be your will. God, Thy will be done. It is not my will, but I will do my best to remember Thy will be done if you need him. AMEN

I embraced him as well as I could and kept repeating, "It's okay, it's okay, I love you, it's okay."

I later realized these were the exact first words I said to Elvis when they laid on him on my chest for the first time, and he cried.

I wanted to play some music and instantly thought of Aretha Franklin's "Amazing Grace." It's a ten-minute version of the song that leaves you feeling as if God is with you. Listening to it, you are transported to a church, a sanctuary filled with song and the Holy Spirit.

Anna arrived as the song was ending. She hadn't been there yet, or seen Nick in person. Nothing could have prepared her for the scene she was walking into, me on his side, holding his hand in my left hand and smoothing his hair with my right. I was wearing a red T-shirt that said MOTHER, black sweatpants, and sneakers. My hair was up in a ponytail, and tears were streaming down my face. But I was calm. There was nothing else I could do, nothing else the doctors could do. So I just stood there, holding on to my husband.

She hugged me tight when she walked in, and we cried together for a long time. She hid her shock at seeing Nick in this state.

"Hey, brother," she said to him, taking his other hand. It had swollen to double its size, and three of the fingertips were now entirely black and blue.

"It's so nice to see you," she said to him. "I've really missed you."

Anna didn't ask me any questions about what had happened or what the doctors had said. She knew I had explained it too many times already, and each time it was more painful to say. She just asked, "What can I do for you, Mandy?"

It was beyond comforting to have her by my side. I hadn't realized how much I had on my shoulders until there was someone else with me, witnessing what I had been witnessing for the past month. She stood with me, and we continued to cry and pray. She held the phone as we called more family members and friends. Hearing their voices and seeing their faces was hard but made us feel less alone.

Dr. Ng came in to check on Nick, and the numbers continued to look bad. He told me that we had an hour, maybe two. He would, of course, do everything he could to keep him alive, but that he didn't think Nick would make it through the night.

As he turned to leave, I said, "Dr. Ng, thank you. I know that you have tried and done everything you could to save my husband."

He could barely look back at me as he left. No one wanted this to be happening.

We sang along with the soft music I was playing, told stories as doctors and nurses moved in and out to check if Nick was still here. We asked how much longer we had, and they said not much. It could be any moment, really.

"Mandy," Anna said, finally breaking down after one of the doctors walked out. "I . . . I can't believe that he isn't going to make it. I never thought he wouldn't make it. I can't believe this is happening."

Together, Anna and I reminded Nick how hard he'd fought, and we thanked him for fighting. We told him how much we loved him and how much Elvis loved him. We said goodbye in every way that we could, and then there was nothing left to do but sit there and wait.

We decided, without actually discussing it, that we didn't want Nick's last moments on this Earth to be sad. We felt like he could hear us. So we told our favorite stories, described our favorite memories. We reminded him and each other of all the good times. We talked about all the beautiful moments, the funny moments, the magical moments. We forced ourselves to smile and laugh and talk about the good days. We still cried. We still felt devastated. But at least by focusing on the light, the room felt less dark.

"Brother," Anna said, "remember when I crashed two thirds of your honeymoon?"

Nick and I had waited until the summer following our wedding to take our honeymoon. We wanted to go to Cape Town and to Kenya for a safari, and that's a trip that requires at least two weeks. Nick was right in the middle of *A Bronx Tale* and couldn't get the time off for both our wedding and an extended honeymoon, so we decided to wait and do the trip the following year.

As the summer approached, other opportunities arose that extended our time away a bit longer. I had been taking an annual trip with family friends to Capri, and they invited Nick along that year. I was also offered a job as the fitness instructor at a wellness retreat in Bali. Our plan was to start in Capri, then travel to Cape Town, to Kenya, and finally end the trip in Bali. The "honeymoon" part of the trip was Africa, but really we celebrated in every destination.

Anna was also on the trip to Capri, and she had been offered a job at the same retreat in Bali, covering social media for the brand. So she started our honeymoon with us in Capri and then met us in Bali for the tail end.

The retreat in Canggu was for women only, but they agreed to let Nick come and do his own thing every day. The "staff," which was just Nick, Anna, and me, had our own villa a few steps from all the guests, so Nick could hang out there to be away from all the ladies. This was okay for the first few days, but he got kind of bored as the week went on. Canggu is a small town, and, without a car, he couldn't easily get around to other parts of the island. He would see us leave every morning and wave goodbye with a sad face. He understood we were working, but he would've obviously preferred for the three of us to be able to hang out instead.

One day the women on the retreat were scheduled to visit a fancy beach club and spend the day enjoying the sun, swimming, and drinking rosé. This was Nick's dream, and we convinced him he should just come, on his own, and be at the same beach club with us.

"I'm sure you can just get your own chair, in your own area, and hang out there. Then maybe I can sneak off and be with you from time to time," I told him. "No one will know that you're there or that you're my husband!"

He was in.

We arrived and got all set up in the front row of the VIP section. This part of the beach club was new, and we were the only people there. Until Nick arrived.

Suddenly, Anna and I noticed an attendant escorting a tall man wearing a swimsuit, an open button-down, and sunglasses over to the VIP section. We poked each other and started laughing hysterically as Nick sprawled out on a sunbed two rows behind us and ordered himself a bottle of rosé.

Nick had been transforming his look at each stop of our honeymoon. In Capri, he was in linen shirts and loafers; in Africa, he had a green safari jacket and an Indiana Jones hat; and after three days in Bali, he was adorned with rings, necklaces, and bracelets, and he was as tan as leather. His hair was wild, and his shirt was always open. He looked like a local.

We had to pretend we didn't know him, even as we walked right by, which made the whole scenario even funnier.

As the day went on, and we got a little tipsy, we got more daring. When no one was looking, Anna passed him an entire platter of left-over sushi that we had ordered, and I sneaked off "to the bathroom" for an hour to meet him at the pool on the other side. We could have just been honest about his being there, and no one would have cared—but keeping it a secret had become so funny we didn't want to.

It meant so much to me that Nick had developed the same kind of relationship with Anna that I had. Anna and I are so alike, it made sense they would get along—but to be able to spend weeks together like this was truly unique. Nick didn't just tolerate Anna's presence, he really wanted her there—often inviting her before I even thought to. We had a great dynamic together, like *Three's Company*.

"I'll never forget you in your full, Bali glory, brother," Anna said to him. "Sprawled out in Finns VIP section in the sunshine, with a bottle of rosé, living your best life."

Hours went by as we talked, and sang, and reminisced, and Nick was still alive. In fact, his numbers were slowly getting better. We kept looking at each other and then at the machines and then back at each other, saying, "Are you seeing this?" Every time the blood pressure got better, Anna and I rejoiced. Every time his oxygen rate climbed a bit higher, we would grab Nick's nurse and say, "Look! He's doing better!"

He was fighting.

We were supposed to leave at nine, when hospital hours were over, but Nick's doctor said we could stay the night if we wanted, likely because he didn't think Nick would make it till morning. I was torn about sleeping there because I had never been away from Elvis for that long, and I was still breastfeeding, but I didn't want to leave Nick's side for a moment. I had to keep going to the ladies' room to squeeze the milk out of my breasts. Todd was on his way from San Francisco. He was going to relieve Rachel around midnight to be with Elvis. It gave me such comfort, knowing he was coming back.

My being there—and Anna's being there—was making a difference. Whatever we were doing, we couldn't stop. So we stayed. They wheeled in a recliner chair for us, and we took turns taking power naps. We continued to call family members and friends, and to play music and tell Nick stories. We had a hospital survival system set up in Nick's room, and Anna and I were the team captains.

His levels were rising. There was no question. Nick continued to improve, little by little. His blood pressure was up in the 70s and 80s even, and his medicines were going down. The oxygen rate was in the high 90s. Anna and I were on to something, or, at least, we believed we were. We had come with a different type of medicine: love, prayer, and support. Nick needed his people by his side. He needed to feel us nearby in order to remember why he needed to fight.

As it got late, we were torn about what to do. Did we stay at the hospital or go home to grab a few hours of sleep and come first thing in the morning? Neither of us knew what was right. The only thing that gave us some comfort was that Nick's numbers were holding steady and looking really good. As it was approaching two thirty, we decided to go home and get a few hours of sleep, shower, and come back when visiting hours started at seven a.m. I had to breastfeed Elvis, or I was going to get an infection. We needed rest, and we knew tomorrow was going to be a long day. We had a job to do!

We hugged Nick, I squeezed his hand, and I gave him the biggest kiss that I could. I thanked his nurse profusely and apologized ahead of time for the number of phone calls I would make throughout the rest of the night to check in. She assured me she would call as soon as possible if anything happened. We felt like zombies, but we stepped out of that room with more adrenaline than we had ever had in our lives. We high-fived in the hallway and hugged and then walked out of the hospital like superheroes who had just saved the planet. We were invigorated, filled with hope. "Thank you, God!" we said. "Thank you! Please, please keep him safe and healthy tonight. You are a miracle worker, Lord!"

They had told me that my husband was going to die that day. That there was nothing else that could be medically done. But against all odds, Nick was still alive.

fourteen

We walked into Brown Bear that night like soldiers returning from battle. Todd's car was in the driveway: Biggie was back.

It was two thirty, Elvis was asleep, and the house was quiet. We went straight to the fridge to see if there was anything we could eat quickly before passing out. Todd appeared from the back room.

"Biggie," we sighed, trying to keep our voices down so as not to wake Elvis.

We both went in at the same time for an enormous hug, putting us back in the same quaranteam huddle we had done just two weeks ago when Todd left. Anna had called him twelve hours before, saying the doctors were certain Nick wouldn't make it through the night. Instead, we told him what had happened, how we stood there watching the numbers rise as we sang, danced, told stories, talked, and called family and friends.

"It had to be us, Biggie," I said. "I think we did it!"

As we got ready for bed, I said to Anna, "I know it's hard to sleep with Petit in the room, but do you think you might be able to sleep in my room tonight?"

"Oh, sister," she replied. "I was already one hundred percent planning on that. I'm not going to leave you alone after a day like today."

I closed my eyes for what felt like five minutes and woke up to sunlight and the delicious smell of something baking. I came out into the kitchen to find Anna removing a tray of hot cookies from the oven and transferring them to racks to cool. They were already at least two dozen stacked on the counter.

"What are you doing?" I laughed.

"Oh, I couldn't sleep," she said. "So I decided to bake. I figured it would be nice to thank all the nurses for yesterday!"

I smiled and nodded.

"I thought I should pack us a lunch, too, so we don't have to leave Nick's room and eat in the gross cafeteria!" She produced two brown paper bags she'd made for us, and I hugged her tight.

We were exhausted but anxious to get back to the hospital. It was too early to call and check on him, but I knew that the lack of a phone call in the middle of the night meant he had made it. He was still alive. We prepared to head into Cedars-Sinai.

So many things were in motion that morning. Yesterday, as we thought Nick was certainly dying, everyone had booked flights to get here to say goodbye to him and to be here for me. Todd's wife and kids were packing up their car and driving down today. My parents were on the way with our best friends from New York. Lesley, Matt, and Amanda were already in transit. Because they're Canadian, they weren't technically allowed into the United States, so getting permission for them had been a huge ordeal that Zach had helped coordinate. They were going to be arriving at LAX at one p.m. Our party of three was about to get twelve new members.

I had sent frantic text messages the night before to Matt Weaver, who immediately came to the rescue, and to a former client of mine who lived down the road in Laurel Canyon. We had two houses at our disposal within a few hours. Both came from complete strangers whom I'd never met, with no strings attached. They didn't want money. They told us the houses were ours for as long as we needed them. All my friends in the Canyon and Elvis's Stroller Buddies—Maddox, Zoe, Erin, and Tom—jumped in to help with drop-offs, babysitting, and groceries.

"Not a single Cordero or Kloots will be paying for a meal," Maddox told us.

He was arranging catered group dinners so we wouldn't have to worry about anything.

"We have a car we aren't using," offered Erin. "The Corderos can use our car for as long as they need it." Looking back, I'm still overwhelmed by how people dropped everything, sprang into action, and went to crazy lengths to help. It was so energizing for me; it felt like we were mobilizing the troops. It was all things I couldn't deal with or even focus on—transportation, accommodations, meals—they all knew that and helped in every way.

We pulled up at Cedars-Sinai, jumped out of the car, and ran in to the registration desk. Anna got through first, and when I got up to the room five minutes later, she was already at Nick's side with his hand in hers.

"You look great, brother; it's so nice to see you," she was saying.

Nick's eyes were wide open.

"Oh, honey! Look at those peepers!" I said. "Hi, Nick, it's Amanda! I love you, honey. We're back! Babes, you did it. We are here all day. Your family is coming today, too! Momsie [Nick's nickname for his mother] will be here in a couple hours! We're going to play you some music, okay?"

We had come up with a plan on the drive here. We were going to be the most positive, encouraging, happy people on the planet that day. We were going to fill his quiet, sad room with music, and dancing, and happiness so that he remembered he had so much joy to live for. We weren't going to let anyone say a negative thing all day.

"Let's do this," I said, connecting my phone to the mini-speaker in

Nick's room. I decided a '60s playlist would be just what Nick would love. I turned it up all the way, pressed play, and we started singing at the top of our lungs, "I know you wanna leave me! But I refuse to let you go."

"This is the perfect song," Anna shouted over the music during a break in the melody.

"I know," I said.

After "Ain't Too Proud to Beg," it was "Ain't No Mountain High Enough," and then "Walk Like a Man."

We got more into it with every song. We sang every word out, we swayed left to right, we spun, we shimmied, we twisted, we snapped our fingers, we shook our heads and tossed our hair. It was seven thirty in the intensive care unit. We were in sweatpants with no makeup on acting like we were in a dance club on a Saturday night. We looked insane.

Nick's nurse was in the anteroom outside his, watching us through the window, utterly confused but smiling.

We didn't let it faze us. We didn't care. We just kept going.

When "I Want to Hold Your Hand" came on, we each took one of Nick's hands and started gently moving them in the way the nurse had shown us was good for his circulation. It was to help the blood flow to his fingers, which were entirely black and swollen now. But it also made it look like he was dancing with us.

Other doctors and nurses from the ICU passed by Nick's room and peered around the corner to see what the hell was going on in room 602. You could undoubtedly hear our music and singing in the other rooms. This is not normal behavior for visitors to the ICU; most people visiting their loved ones probably spent the time crying. But not us; what good would that do for anyone? We weren't acting normal, but we didn't care. We were delirious, hysterical, and high on adrenaline. We weren't stopping unless they made us.

"Yep! The Kloots sisters have arrived on the sixth floor," I yelled, laughing.

"That's right," Anna said. "This floor could use some pep!"

We realized how quiet and sad the whole floor was. So many patients were without any visitors because of COVID, just lying there alone in the quiet. It was awful.

"We should dance over to some of the other rooms," I said. "Bring the other people some music!"

"Hey, that's a brilliant idea," Anna said. "When this is all over, we should do this, Mands! We should volunteer at the hospital once a week, come visit patients in the ICU and sing and dance for them! We can call ourselves the Patient Pep Squad!"

As we did our routine, Nick's levels continued to rise. We cheered and danced bigger every time one of his levels improved. "Keep those numbers rising, Nick, you're doing it, babes!" I said to him. The doctors and Nick's nurse couldn't beg to differ. He was looking good, very alert, and his numbers were high and steady.

Anna put on the next song, and we sang, "Your love, liftin' me higher."

His eyes were wide open; he knew I was there. He was fighting; I could see it. He was fighting for his life, for Elvis, for me.

Hours flew by like minutes. The doctors and nurses came in to check on him and were mystified.

"Hi, Dr. Ng," I shouted over the music when he entered. "Look at our guy! Look at his levels!"

Dr. Ng looked utterly confused and enthralled at the same time.

"There's no explaining this," Dr. Ng said. "I would have bet everything he was not going to make it through the night. This is a miracle, Amanda. I . . . I can't explain it. If things stay like this, I don't know. We could be okay."

Anna and I high-fived triumphantly.

"When is his family arriving?" Dr. Ng asked.

The Corderos had landed and were on their way. Matt Weaver had just called Anna; he had picked them up from the airport and they were on the way to the hospital. Anna went to meet them when they arrived so that they wouldn't get lost in the maze of Cedars.

"I know hugs aren't allowed, but desperate times call for desperate measures," she said, embracing Lesley. "Did you get in okay?"

Lesley arrived at the hospital, cool, calm, and collected. She blew me away with her composure and strength when she walked into the room and saw Nick for the first time. They had all had a long journey here but had gotten off the plane to the news that Nick was stable, his levels having improved. We weren't out of the woods, but we were making progress. They had expected to arrive and find him already gone. The fact that he was still alive was reason enough to rejoice.

We weren't all allowed in the room at the same time, so Anna and I left and let Nick's family have some time alone with him. I knew they were seeing this all for the first time; it was going to be a shock for them to be in the room. They absolutely needed their alone time. I also knew how much seeing them would lift Nick's spirits even more. His mother and family meant the world to him. He called his mom every day; he adored his baby sister, Amanda; and he had a new-father bond with his younger brother, whose wife had had a baby girl just a few days before Elvis was born. The Corderos are all about family, and now Nick had his by his side. I was so happy for him and for them.

We went outside the ICU doors to a little waiting area, and there was no one else there, not even a guard. Anna and I slouched into chairs and passed out. We needed to rest up for round two of the Patient Pep Squad.

We took another shift when the Corderos went for a lunch break. Nick was still alert, like he was waiting to see what other surprises were in store for him. I knew the doctors wanted to see progress, so I tried for anything I could. By five p.m., a mere fourteen hours after they told me he had maybe an hour left to live, I had Nick tracking. I asked him to follow my commands, and he did.

"Look left, look right, look up, look down," I said. Then I held out my finger and asked him to follow it up, down, left, and right. Then I told him, "Babe, give me a big smile. Come on, honey, smile for me."

The corner of his upper lip lifted up as much as he could to show me he was trying to smile.

My heart exploded, I burst into happy tears. I was told the best option fourteen hours ago was to put him in comfort care, and now he was tracking and smiling.

Around six p.m., we left the hospital to meet my parents, who had arrived with our friends from New York, Saskia, Hugh, and their two daughters. The houses were being made ready, so everyone convened that night at Brown Bear to have dinner and put together a plan. We all would stay outside and try to keep as much distance as possible, but we had all been privately quarantining for months now, so we were certain we didn't have COVID. Everyone thought they would arrive under very different circumstances, so our evening became a celebration. We also hadn't seen each other since January, and it was now the end of May. Just to see the people you loved was so special.

When Anna and I pulled into the driveway, everyone was already there. We walked through the doors like superheroes, yet again announcing to everyone "He's stable!" as they cheered. Then we went into the details of our pep squad routine, reenacting our spectacle.

"We're going to go right back there tomorrow and do the same thing," I said.

Everyone settled into their new homes that night. My parents and brother were a ten-minute drive from me near The Flats of Beverly Hills. Lesley, Matt, and Amanda were literally down the street in Laurel Canyon. It couldn't have been a better setup.

Anna and I offered to take the morning shift again to allow the Corderos to get some sleep. We got to Cedars first thing, passed through security with minimal trouble, and headed into Nick's room.

Yesterday it had been "Sixties on Six," since Nick was on the sixth floor.

Today we had decided it would be "Michael Jackson Monday!"

Nick loved Michael's music, and he had so many albums that we could sing every word to, so we knew we would be able to do a full performance.

We got on either side of his bed right away and started our singing ... "Just beat it (beat it), beat it (beat it), No one wants to be defeated."

There we were again, day two, the pep squad singing and dancing with Nick.

We were so invigorated and genuinely having so much fun being there, filling his room with happiness, that each song brought us more smiles and moves. The nurses, now used to our crazy methods, kept walking by and looking into the room, giving us a thumbs-up or telling us, "We love the music, keep it up!" During "Billie Jean," we saw through the window a tall male nurse doing the moonwalk down the hall. We had the whole floor on our side now, and Nick's levels were rising with the beat.

In the afternoon, the Corderos came, while Anna and I checked on our parents and Todd's family. They had Elvis for the day, and the house they were staying in had a beautiful, big pool. It was a warm, sunny day in LA, so we found them all swimming and having fun together when we arrived. My family is always so happy to be together that we can appreciate being with one another, even during difficult, stressful times.

Anna and I went back for the late-night shift that evening, planning to stay until they kicked us out. We continued to sing and tell Nick stories, and we played him recordings of Elvis cooing and making little sounds that we had on our phones. He really responded to hearing Elvis, so I had our friends make a CD on a constant loop to play in his room. We FaceTimed with everyone again so that they could see his progress and cheer him on, and we could tell this really helped Nick; I knew that it encouraged him.

That evening I got a phone call and walked outside of Nick's room to take it. Shockingly, it was Jennifer Love Hewitt on the line. She had been following Nick's story and had posted several stories singing, praying, supporting, doing anything and everything she could. She was so kind. It was as if we had known each other for years.

"How are you doing?" she asked. "What can I do for you? I reached out to some of my friends; there are so many people who want to help you.

"I have secured meals for you and your family two nights a week from my friend's food delivery. I also have diapers for you! A one-year supply. I talked to Jennifer Garner, too, and she's going to give you baby food from her new line. What are you doing for Elvis's first birthday?" she asked.

"Oh gosh," I replied, so overwhelmed by her kindness. "I don't know. I feel so bad. I haven't had time to think of anything. Anna said she'd take charge of planning it all."

"Okay!" she exclaimed. "I've got it under control. All I need Anna to do is pick a theme, and I will take care of the decor, tables, food, and desserts!"

I hung up the phone and walked back into Nick's room, looking at Anna with my mouth hanging open.

"I think she might be the kindest person on the planet. Also, I can't believe I just talked to Jennifer Love Hewitt!" We had watched the movie *Can't Hardly Wait* a million times.

I told Anna everything she had offered and how she wouldn't take no for an answer.

"Let's pick a theme for Elvis's birthday then, sister," she said. "We love a theme! How about a 1950s drive-in?" We ordered saddle shoes on Amazon that night.

Dr. Ng came in before leaving for the night to check on Nick and talk to us. I showed him a video I took of Nick tracking, smiling. He was impressed and, I could tell, happy. He didn't want to lose Nick either. He had to break the bad news that now that Nick was "stable" again, we had to cut down our visits. So I would be the only one allowed into the hospital. Letting us all in had been a big bending of the rules, a risk they allowed because Nick was so critical and because his family had flown in. Now, though, we needed to get back to hospital protocol. It was heartbreaking for Anna and the Corderos, but we all understood. We were just thankful that I would still be allowed to be with Nick. That someone could be by his side.

They kicked us out at midnight that night, which we understood. It was a lot easier to leave Cedars now that I knew I'd be allowed back in without question, and now that Nick was stable and aware.

"We're going to let you rest now, honey," I said as we left.

Anna said. "It's goodbye from me for a bit—but don't worry, I'll be back. You blow me away, Nick. You're a rock star. No one's ever done what you just did! I am in awe!"

When we got home, the exhaustion of spending the last two days at the hospital, having all the new visitors, and being a mom set in. I was in a fog and felt so torn about being at home and not at the hospital. It was always a struggle to feel okay wherever I was. At home, Elvis needed me, and I wanted to be with him. At the hospital, Nick needed me, and I wanted to be with him. It was a painful choice, but easy at the same time. As the only person allowed in the hospital—being there became my full-time job. Little ak took over for me with Elvis the next morning and for the next two weeks. Todd took supervising my house renovations.

I pulled on my sweats, slicked my hair into a bun, and off I went back to Cedars-Sinai for day three of keeping Nick alive.

As I went to the hospital, I had a new plan now that I would be there alone. People had told me that if I could get into the hospital, I should try to lie beside him. Also, ever since I'd connected with Steph the healer, and she had correctly identified the injured spot in Nick's brain, I had been in close contact with her. She was incredible, relaying what she was getting from her sessions with Nick. It was in one of my recent exchanges with her that she'd said something honestly scary because it was something Nick would say to me all the time.

"Nick," she told me, "is remembering how much he loves the feeling of having Elvis asleep on his chest." I needed to do something about that.

I tried very hard from the beginning to sleep train Elvis. I was stern about bedtime and naps and making sure Elvis slept alone in his crib. Elvis had a nap every day around nine a.m., when I often taught a fitness class. I would tell Nick that he just had to put Elvis down for his nap and he would sleep the whole time I was gone. We went over songs to sing and things to do, and I would leave for Bandier, hoping he would adhere to the rules.

When I got back from class, I'd open the door and hear no noise in the cabin. *Yes,* I'd think, *he did it!* But then I'd walk into the bedroom, and there they were: Nick lying on the bed and Elvis passed out on his chest with a lovey. I would want to be angry because he wasn't following the rules. But they looked so cute, all I could do each time I found them this way was take a photo.

Nick would always defend his actions, saying, "What am I supposed to do? He's so cuddly, and he just passes out on me! It's the best feeling!"

As a parent, you make plans for how you're going to take advantage of nap time, or how you'll create a schedule to keep your child on. But then one thing leads to another, and twenty minutes later you've become a body pillow for a six-month-old. You know that it's a bad habit, and yet you can't help yourself, because you also know that these moments are special. Plus, if you move, you risk waking up your baby!

So much of parenting is about these plans we make that life, or reality, interferes with. As parents, we often find it hard to enjoy the moments we're given, because we lie there thinking about the things we should be doing instead. I tried my hardest to stick to the plan—but Nick was always able to enjoy these moments with Elvis. It was his new version of Fantasyland.

When Steph told me, "Nick misses that weight on his chest and holding Elvis," it brought me to instant tears.

I turned those words over as I was en route to Cedars-Sinai. The idea of crawling into bed with him sounded impossible; there were so many wires and tubes, and the bed was small, especially for two very tall people. But it was worth a try. I wanted to lie down next to Nick, put my weight against him, and connect with him. It was just me here today.

Once I arrived, I started my routine. I always said a prayer first thing, thanking God that Nick was still here and asking for a good day with more good news. I then picked a playlist and turned on the tunes. I went with Laurel Canyon classics and started telling him the story of buying our home and then fantasizing about living there when he got out of the hospital.

The next time the nurse walked in, I got brave enough to ask my question: Could I possibly lie next to him in the hospital bed?

"Oh, sure, Amanda," she said. "I think we can make that happen! Let me get someone to help me slide him over. I think you should lie on his right side because there will be more room from the amputation."

It is amazing to watch nurses work, especially ICU nurses. They move around so freely and confidently when, to an outsider, it appears like everything in the room should be stamped FRAGILE. Two of them used his blankets to slide his body over to the left side of his bed so that I could shimmy onto the right side. One nurse positioned the cords and tubes in such a way that I couldn't disturb them. I got into position—the position I would take if we were sleeping in bed together at home—my head right at his chest, my right leg over his left, and my right arm over his body. She tucked us in and said, "Hold one minute, and I'll be right back." She returned a moment later with a fresh warm blanket, the final layer to our cozy, new bed.

I couldn't hold back the tears; they poured out of me. I had missed this, had missed Nick so much. I hadn't been able to hold my husband in months.

"I'll give you some alone time, Amanda. I'll dim the lights and close the curtain and be right outside and only come in if I need to check something. Otherwise, just relax and be with him. I am so glad we could set this up," the nurse said.

Through my tears, I thanked her profusely.

I switched the music to Ella Fitzgerald, one of our favorite dinner playlists, and tried my best to pull it together. "Dream a little dream of me . . ."

It felt like we were transported back in time. I closed my eyes. There in the dark, I could forget for a moment *where* we were. *How* we were.

I heard machines go off and people come in and out periodically, but otherwise, I slept, and so did Nick. I wasn't Elvis, but I was hoping I had fulfilled the weight on his chest that he was missing. I slept, holding my man in my arms, head on his chest, as Ella sang. It was absolutely perfect and something I will never, ever forget.

I woke up hours later. Nick's eyes were wide open.

"Oh, babes, that was wonderful," I said to him. "It felt so good to lie next to you and sleep. I love you, honey."

I hadn't told Steph what time I was going to the hospital or what I was planning on doing, but as I started messaging with her, she said to me, "I felt a powerful love presence this morning, Amanda, like around eleven a.m."

I was in disbelief: that was precisely when I climbed into bed with him.

Any time I came home from the hospital, I had to strip and shower right away. All the clothes had to go straight into the washing machine. I would text Anna or Todd as I was pulling in the driveway so they knew to hide Elvis until I was ready because he would scream if he saw me. But once I was clean, I could sneak up behind him.

"I missed you! How are you, honey?" I'd asked. He would give me the biggest smile and then go right for my shirt.

"Oh, okay, you want a boob? I got ya, give me a second."

Within moments I was in a chair breastfeeding. My lunch had to wait, even though I hadn't eaten all day. Luckily, Diana, Todd's wife, had been cooking and had a lunch buffet ready to go.

At three p.m., I got on Instagram Live to sing. My whole family joined in with me as I sang into a Bluetooth microphone that had mysteriously shown up in a package one day. It was tough to go live a lot of days because I couldn't say that I had been in the hospital to see Nick. I couldn't let on how critical he was. I had to act! Fortunately, I am an actress, and I put on a brave face, as if I'd been at home all day and Nick was doing okay. I felt so guilty seeing people say, "I hope you can go see him soon," or "They should let you in the hospital." I couldn't say I was already inside, but I didn't want to lie, so I just didn't address it.

I took a quick nap in the sun, and then at four, I went back to Cedars. That evening, my family was outside, having a huge BBQ feast that Maddox had arranged for us. I FaceTimed them from the hospital with Nick so we could be there with everyone. It was so special for Nick to see everyone together. It was his dream that everyone we loved would move to LA. He would always say to me, "If we go there, everyone will come. You'll see!"

"We all came for you, Nick," they shouted. Everyone was so ecstatic about his turnaround. It really felt as if his survival was certain at this point. He had proven how strong he was, how hard he was willing to fight.

Well, he was right. They had all come here.

Before I left the hospital that night, I said a prayer with Nick. *Lord, please keep him safe through the night. Send your angels to be by his side. Send your Holy Spirit down and cover him with your glory. AMEN.*

The next morning, I received a message from Steph. She had just come out of a session and got the sense that Nick was deciding whether he wanted to fight anymore or not. She wrote, "He knows life won't be the same for him ever again, and I could feel he was scared. He feels that if he fights and survives, what kind of husband will he be able to be? Will he be able to work, provide for his family? What kind of Dad would he be to Elvis with the limitations to his body after the strokes? Would he be able to hold his son even?"

This rocked me to my core. It sounded like exactly what Nick would have said if he could have talked to me. This insight into his headspace made me so sad. I knew that he had to surrender and trust God and be okay with his new body, his new way of life. But Nick didn't have my faith, or any faith at all really. The idea of waking up and not living the same life would scare him, and I could understand why he was second-guessing fighting for it. If he could speak, I bet he would say, "Maybe you would be better off, Amanda, if I wasn't here. I'll be a burden to you if I never get stronger. You're young and should have a life." I could hear him saying it. Nick was the kind of person who always saw both sides and could argue them. It infuriated me because in an argument, he would get me to agree with him on his point, but then he would instantly begin defending the other perspective. I drove to the hospital on a mission to convince him there was only one way to look at things this time, and for once, at least, I knew he couldn't argue the other side.

"Hi, honey," I said when I got to his room.

"I have to talk to you, because I know you're struggling with this. I know you're thinking you'll be a burden and won't be a good dad to Elvis. But I'm going to argue the other side now: you will be the most incredible role model for him, Nick. He'll know that his dad defied all odds, that his dad is a fighter, and he will look at you in awe, honey. He will be so proud that Nick Cordero is his dad. You have to trust in that.

"You're right that your life will not be the same, but God has a plan for you, honey. You have so many people praying for you, people who have never prayed in their lives are praying for you. You are helping so many people to have faith, and everyone is rooting for your Code Rocky! So *you* have to have faith now. *You* have to root for your Code Rocky, and believe that the new life God has in store for you is going to be more amazing than you can even fathom right now.

"I had a vision the other day that you were playing the Super Bowl halftime show. It was the first Super Bowl after COVID, and they brought you out to sing "Live Your Life." The whole stadium was singing with you, on their feet, cheering you on. Elvis and I were there watching. You were doing it, babes! I see it. I believe in you, and that God is protecting you.

"The doctors told me you weren't going to make it; they said there was nothing more medically they could do. But I sat here next to you and prayed, and you survived; you're still here. That is God's work, Nick. He's keeping you here for a reason. I know you don't believe in

God, but you have to trust Him now. Yes, this will change us, but you have to believe it will change us for the better. I'm right here by your side, every step of the way! I'm not giving up, and I'm not leaving. So get any ideas out of your head that you're not wanted or not needed, because you are!"

When I was done, I could see in his eyes that he saw my point. If he could have spoken, he would have said, *Amanda, you're right.*

At the end of that week, our family and friends decided to go back home, and Nick's siblings, Matt and Amanda, booked their return flight a couple of days out. We had one last evening all together, and some of Elvis's Stroller Buddies insisted on ordering us my favorite pizza from Blackbird. We tried to stop them—they were already doing so much for us—but they were insistent.

Blackbird is a Chicago-style deep-dish pizzeria on Melrose that Nick and I found while we lived in LA during my pregnancy. We loved it so much that we would sometimes go twice a week, order a large, and eat it all. I convinced myself that it wasn't bad for me, since I was eating for two. The last time we ordered from Blackbird was in March when quarantine hit. Nick was already sick and unable to get off the couch, but it was before we knew he had COVID. I thought ordering Blackbird would jolt his appetite. Unfortunately, it didn't, he barely had two bites of his piece, and I ate the rest. I couldn't blame it on Elvis that time.

It was a Sunday evening, so before dinner we all met on the street for Laurel Canyon Community Choir. When I pulled up, our #teamNick party included fifteen people, making for the best turnout choir practice ever had! Todd had his arm around Diana, and Oliver and Hudson were snapping photos in the street with their Instax. My mom was hand in hand with Anna, who had Elvis strapped to her in his baby carrier. Lesley was next to Matt and Amanda. I headed down the hill;

took in the whole, magical scene in the street; and felt so blessed to have family members and friends like these: people who would pause their lives and fly across the country to be here with me. There is something wonderful about singing "You've Got a Friend" and "Our House," on the very streets where those songs were written, while surrounded by your loved ones.

Back at the house, we dug into pizza and cozied into our chairs to watch a movie. That night, to go with our pizza party, Jennifer Love Hewitt had sent an outdoor cinema service to set up a giant screen, lounge chairs, and a popcorn machine in the driveway of Brown Bear so we could have a family movie night. It was the perfect last hurrah to celebrate the miraculous turnaround and the time we had been able to spend together. We had our choice of anything, and we decided on *My Cousin Vinny* because it's so funny. It's a family classic and one of my dad's favorite movies. I was kind of in a blur as we watched. I couldn't pay much attention to the movie, but I do remember how nice it was to just sit outside, on a warm night, surrounded by the people whom I loved most in the world, and I'll never forget the wonderful sound of everyone's laughter.

fifteen

It's difficult to notice the change of seasons in Los Angeles, since it's seventy-two degrees and sunny no matter the month. But when I was a New Yorker, Memorial Day marked the official start of summer, and everyone celebrated it. Nick and I loved to flee the city for the summer holiday weekends, even if it was just to go a few hours upstate. We would rent an Airbnb with a pool and a yard so we could play house.

A few weeks after Elvis was born we took our first family trip up to Hudson, New York, with my parents and sisters. We were used to packing a duffel bag for a weekend away and taking the train, but now we had a baby. As new parents, we were so afraid to forget something critical that we loaded an entire rental car with his toys, swaddles, diapers, and devices, despite planning to be away for only forty-eight hours. Nick's patience making several runs back up the apartment for all the things we realized we forgot while loading the car was shocking. He didn't complain once. He really wanted this trip to happen.

When we got to Hudson, he practically skipped through the aisles of the suburban-style grocery store, filling the cart with things I'd never seen him once eat in the three years I'd known him, and enough beer and wine to throw a frat party. He loaded it all in the fridge when we got to the house, and then spent the rest of the afternoon intermittently floating in the pool on an inflatable avocado and jumping out to change diapers. After grilling steaks with my dad, eating Anna's homemade peach pie, and looking up at the stars, Nick and I cozied up on the couch, my head in his lap and Elvis lying across my belly. The getaway had been a huge success, and Nick was so happy to be out of Manhattan, getting a glimpse of what life in a real home of our own would be like. He wore a particular expression when he was content like this—his lips upturned in a big grin and a visible gleam in his eye. When I saw him like that, I just knew that everything was right in his world. As I sat next to him in the hospital on Memorial Day, I thought about that smile and how I missed it.

He had survived the impossible last week, but the infection in his lungs was not going away. I had dedicated every spare moment I had over the last week to researching anything that might help him. Each night, I combed through direct messages on Instagram, checked emails, and spent hours on the phone with anyone willing to talk to me. At that time, I was so desperate for something that could save Nick that no matter how crazy or unconventional the idea seemed, I clung to a shred of hope that it could work—and there was no shortage of treatment ideas. I looked into every single one, grasping for some reason it could be the answer. When something sounded reasonable, or possible, or had worked for someone with a similar case, I'd dive into research and use every resource I had to learn more. That was how I learned about a man named Edward Pierce, a Broadway set designer who was the first to receive a new treatment from a company called Pluristem Therapeutics. It had developed a procedure that involved injecting a patient with placental stem cells; the idea was to stimulate the body to regenerate and repair tissue that had been damaged by COVID. Through the Broadway community, I was able to talk to Edward directly just hours after I learned about him. He had spent forty-six days on a ventilator and was now home with his wife, COVID free. He told me they had tried the

Pluristem treatment as a Hail Mary pass because his doctors were out of ideas for him. He firmly believed it was the stem cells that saved his life. That was all I needed to hear to begin looking into whether we might be able to try it for Nick. I wanted to learn as much as I could before presenting it to Dr. Ng.

My morning call with the nurses was a bit tough, because the visitation rules had changed yet again. I was still the only one allowed in, but now I was allowed in for just four hours each day. Although we had proven that my being there helped him, and that he declined each time they restricted my visits, I understood the hospital's rules. It was frustrating, though. My only comfort was that I believed my pep talk had convinced Nick to keep fighting. He had seen his family; he had heard their voices. I knew that the contact he had with everyone he loved had reminded him how much he needed to fight for this life.

The nurse told me that he was going to have a busy morning. They wanted to do another bronch sweep to clean out his lungs. No matter how often they did this, there was always a lot of mucus to come out. "Too much," they said each time. Dr. Ng suggested that they prone Nick again. They had done this in the early days of his time in the ICU, and it had helped get oxygen to his lungs. Nick was to lie on his belly for sixteen hours to open up his breathing passages, which would hopefully help his pH levels get better, and in turn get him out of acidosis.

We FaceTimed with him that morning, but he was so tired he didn't even make eye contact with me once. Because of the sweep, I had to wait until a little later in the morning to go visit him. The time allowed me to film a morning workout for my subscription series. I had to upload a video the next day, and this was my chance to get work done for my business, so Anna took Elvis on a stroll and I had the hour to myself.

On her now daily walks with Elvis, she would do a French lesson aloud—getting some practice in while hoping Elvis would pick up a word or two. "Just getting him ready for his eventual visit to Paris," she always said. He was eleven months old but not yet walking or saying a peep. He had learned how to clap for himself, give kisses if we asked, and pull himself up onto his feet, but not a single word yet. I had given up on sleep training completely, pulling him into bed with Anna and me the second he let out his first cry and cuddling him for the rest of the night. We were getting an average of four to five hours of solid rest a night, but nothing could be done about it. Truth be told, we both loved his cuddles as much as he loved not being alone in his crib. Elvis developed much faster when he got to spend time with my family every afternoon, suddenly around ten people for part of the day, instead of just Anna and me, and you could see the difference in him.

When I finally got to the hospital that day, Nick was about to be proned. He was still on his back and looked tired. Bronch sweeps really took everything out of him. So while I waited, I was on the phone with Edward Pierce's wife, asking more questions about the Pluristem treatment. Dr. Welch was in and out of Nick's room, checking on his progress. When I got his attention, I brought up Pluristem and told him what I'd learned. Dr. Welch sat and listened and then, to my surprise, said to me, "In my opinion, it's time to start doing everything we can safely do to see if it helps his immune system fight the sepsis. We are running out of time . . ."

I couldn't help but think that maybe this could be our Hail Mary pass. I mentioned Edward's case to both Dr. John and Dr. Ng, and they both agreed to research the information with me. They saw the logic behind why this could work: we weren't trying to fight COVID anymore; that infection was gone. We were now trying to repair the damage that COVID had done to his lungs, and that's exactly what stem cells do. It had worked for Edward; it could work for Nick. But in talking to Edward's doctor, Dr. Ng discovered that Edward had spiked a fever after receiving the treatment. His health declined a bit before he got better. If that were to happen to Nick, it would be detrimental. We couldn't afford any backward steps at this point. Dr. Ng also reminded me that every case, every patient, is different. There was no way of knowing if it would even work for Nick, and they felt there wasn't enough research. I understood their point, but we needed a Hail Mary, and I wasn't ready to give up on this yet. In a time where nothing made sense to me, anything that did—even a bit—gave me hope.

That week, the doctor started Nick on a high dose of vitamin C and steroids, which were being used to treat other patients recovering from COVID. There was little to no research that either of these would make a difference, but it was helpful to me to know that something new was being done. I was asked to step out of the room, while ten doctors and nurses went through the process of flipping Nick into the proning position. I was fascinated by how they could do this with all the wires connected to machines, Nick's trach, and his heavy, lifeless six-foot-five-inch body. It took about ten minutes, and I listened from the anteroom to all of the distinct instructions. I was in constant awe of how incredible the doctors and nurses were, how they knew what to do every time.

In the proning position, I couldn't hold his hands because they were too close to his head. His head was entirely to one side, and drool would seep out of his mouth, soaking a towel that was propping up his face. I tried to maneuver through the wires but feared that I'd mess something up. So I awkwardly reached for his head and played with his hair. It was hard to feel like I was doing anything, but it didn't matter; I just wanted him to know that he wasn't alone.

I sat there, trying to come up with an activity to do while passing the day with Nick, when a nurse came in and handed me a massive pile of mail. I couldn't believe what I saw: handwritten multiple-page letters, get-well cards, and gifts. We were in a pandemic, yet people had found a way to get cards and mail them to Nick. I opened each letter, card, and package and read to Nick from his stack of fan mail. The innate kindness of people from all over the world, hoping and praying for him to get his Code Rocky, was astounding. I saved every single one, brought them home so my family and Lesley could read them, and then put them into a big bin of memorabilia Anna had started for me. It was full of all the things that we knew Nick would want to see when he left the hospital, and that Elvis would want to read when he was old enough.

Anna and Todd sent me videos each day of Elvis playing with his cousins, swimming or playing games, which made me so happy. In one he was sitting on a yoga mat, playing with my jump rope. He was laughing so hard and moving his arms up and down, holding the handles. I never felt terrible being away from him when I saw how much he was enjoying being with my family; I just felt thankful that he was too young to understand what was going on. I had started to record Elvis's laughs and babbling so I could play them for Nick at the hospital. I wanted him to hear Elvis's voice so he would remember him and feel connected. I stayed with Nick until I was told to leave or needed to go home to feed Elvis and put him to bed. When I came home, I sneaked inside and took my hot shower. Then I put on my brave face and a smile and went to grab my son—right from my one man to my other.

My family members had decided not to leave after all, so we had to figure out where everyone would live. The home they had been given for that week was not a long-term option. So Diana took on the project of finding us a new place to go. We needed a lot of space to accommodate all of us, and unfortunately, in Los Angeles, space doesn't come cheap. As we searched for something we could afford, we were also hoping to find something big enough for Anna, Elvis, and me to move into as well. I had been occupying Zach's guesthouse since September, and I felt as if I was overstaying my welcome—though he never once made me feel that way and insisted that I could stay as long as I needed.

Meanwhile, the Corderos were having their own dilemma. They were still not allowed in the hospital and were growing frustrated. They had flown all the way from Canada and wanted to be by Nick's side.

Nick's siblings were planning to leave soon. Matt, Nick's brother, had a baby girl at home who was Elvis's age. When he returned to Canada, he would have to quarantine for two weeks before he would be able to see her. Nick's sister, Amanda, runs a boutique and had to get back to work. Lesley was debating whether or not to leave and return when Nick got out of the hospital. But she worried about traveling, and about getting back into the country. No one really knew what to do. I had told the doctors over the weekend that Nick's family would be leaving and begged the staff to allow the Corderos to visit one last time to say goodbye. Luckily, a status meeting was scheduled for the morning of May 26, the day before they planned to leave. They would meet with the doctors one last time, and then be allowed to visit with Nick.

It was daunting each time one of these meetings happened. I hated sitting in that cold, desolate little room as the doctors delivered their bad news. I don't know how they're able to do these meetings day after day, while remaining emotionless and detached. I'm not blaming them—it's their job, and they're amazing at it. It's just that my nature is to maintain a glass-half-full outlook, and the ICU doctors seemed to look at me as if there wasn't even a glass there at all. They started the meeting by acknowledging Nick's progress from last week, but went on to stress that his infection was not getting better, despite the heavy antibiotics he was on, and it had grown into a major concern. They repeated that each time he got a new infection, his overall health dipped. If the infection eventually cleared, he didn't fully return to where he'd been before it happened. He was losing ground. The high-dose steroids were helping but not enough. "We are out of ideas," they said.

"Well," I said with a smile, not missing a beat, "then let's talk placentas!" Dr. Ng smirked, and the rest of the team looked at me like I was nuts.

I argued, "I know I sound crazy—you're looking at me like I am—but I don't care! This is my husband's life! I will bring every crazy idea to the table until there are no more to bring." I spoke passionately and presented all my research on the Pluristem treatment. But to my despair, they all shook their heads and laid out their arguments against this plan. They had made calls and done their research and weren't on board. *The cases weren't the same. Pluristem wasn't FDA approved. There wasn't enough research. It could backfire and cause further stress and damage to Nick's body.* I had invested so much hope into this idea, being told no was a hard pill for me to swallow. I was desperate for solutions to help him, and so out of my mind with grief that I could see only the possible reward, not the risk. My biggest point had been: "What do we have to lose here?" But the doctors reminded me that we had *everything* to lose. In Nick's fragile state, we couldn't afford to take any risks. I realized they were right. It was not an option, and I needed to move on. There was nothing to do but stay hopeful; Nick was too young to give up on. We had just seen him survive the impossible last week. Dr. Ng assured me that they were doing everything to help Nick—looking into every option—and deep down I knew that was true. But it didn't stop me from going home and spending hours researching the next possibility.

This was the first, but not last, grand idea I discovered, researched exhaustively, and pitched to the doctors . . . only to have them dismiss it. I understand now, and I did then, that these new treatments are often looked at by medical professionals as trendy, experimental, or holistic. I was working with a top team of doctors at one of the world's best hospitals, and I never felt like I knew better than they did. But I also couldn't ignore the DMs, emails, and suggestions coming my way, and I wasn't afraid to look stupid presenting things to the team. It gave me something to hope for, and it made me feel like I was doing everything I could, instead of just accepting that my husband was dying. My theory in life is that no one knows everything, and collaboration often is the key to success.

When we finally got to Nick's room, he looked worse than we had ever seen him. The ICU is often one step forward, two steps back. We had all been so encouraged just a few days ago, and now it felt like all that progress had been lost, and we were in a worse place than before. We never let Nick feel that, or see that, though. We always talked to one another as if he could hear us because we believed that he could. If we were in his room, only encouraging things were coming out of our mouths. The Corderos told him childhood stories to bring back happy memories. Nick loved retelling stories. They laughed a lot, holding his hands and being by his side. Lesley would say to him, "I'll love you forever, I'll like you for always," which is a line from a children's book she had read to him when he was a little boy. She'd been saying that to him his whole life.

As we were preparing to leave, Dr. Welch appeared in the hallway and pulled us into the small anteroom off Nick's room to talk to us. We had already finished our meeting, so this second—impromptu—one caught us off guard. These talks were so emotionally draining that to have two in one day was a lot. But he knew Nick's family was planning to leave, and I think he saw this as his last opportunity to talk to them. Dr. Welch never sugarcoated anything.

"It is time you face reality and accept the facts," he began, talking slowly and sternly.

"His lungs are destroyed from COVID. There are giant holes that will never heal. When I do a bronch sweep on him, he looks up at me, and I see pain in his eyes. They haunt me for the rest of the night. No treatment is going to help him now. He is never going to leave this hospital. He is never going to make it to rehab. He is going to die here. It is time to move Nick to comfort care."

We had to bring over a chair for Lesley to sit in. I had grown used to Dr. Welch's bluntness, so I wasn't as affected as Lesley, but no one had said these words before, not with this degree of certainty. It was the first time the humaneness of this situation was pushed on us, and we were made to feel like we were keeping Nick alive for us, instead of for him. Dr. Welch presented the option of moving Nick to comfort care like it was an order, not a suggestion, and his words were so exact and brutal, they left us all stunned. We walked out of the hospital that night speechless. With his words in mind, Lesley decided she was not leaving California. Matt and Amanda were supposed to fly out the following morning, but they decided to push their flights back another few days to see how things developed. The hospital agreed to allow me to keep visiting, but only me. So for the next two days, I went to be by Nick's side alone. The stress and uncertainty had mounted in all of us.

On May 28, the riots and protests broke out in Los Angeles in response to the murder of George Floyd. Anna and I watched the news each day with growing sadness at what had happened and fear about what would result. At three that afternoon, protesters started marching from the Santa Monica Police Station at 333 Olympic Drive to an LAPD substation in Venice. This first protest appeared peaceful, but we saw on the news reports of violence in other cities around the United States and grew more scared. My parents and Todd's family were moving that week to the new place in Studio City, so I would leave the hospital in the evening and we would all have dinner together at their new house. I would catch everyone up on what the doctors had said, how Nick was, and how I was feeling. Then Anna and I would drive home to Brown Bear and put Elvis to bed. Since Nick had survived and the family arrived, we had been in this little routine. There was no progress but no huge setbacks either. I actually enjoyed days of no news. But on the morning of the May 29, the phone rang. I had already called the hospital at six thirty for my usual morning check-in, and everything had been stable. I was supposed to go in around noon.

I sprang up and answered the call; it was Dr. Welch.

"Amanda, how quickly can you all get here?" he asked.

My whole body seized up, frozen with a rush of anxiety.

"Wha-what?" I asked. "Why?"

"Nick is very bad. You should come; so should Nick's family. You should all get here as quickly as you can. Noon might be too late. He might not make it to noon."

"What?" I repeated. "I just spoke to the nurse. What happened?"

"He took a bad turn. Can you bring Elvis with you to say goodbye?" he asked. "If it were me, I'd want to see my son."

I had begged, *pleaded*, to be allowed to bring Elvis into the room for weeks, even if it was for just a minute. Every single time I'd asked I'd gotten a stern "no" in response. It was too dangerous for him, which I understood. Now I was suddenly allowed? I was so flustered that I could barely speak. Elvis was on a walk in the Canyon with Anna. They had left a while before.

"Of course, yes, but . . . is he allowed? They have always said no," I said.

"I'm not sure; I'll ask and call you right back."

They were always so vague on the phone, never giving me any details, which led me to assume the worst. A nurse had told me Nick was stable just an hour ago. What could possibly have happened? But that was the thing—in the ICU, a patient's status can change instantaneously, and for Nick, it did—time and time again.

Panicking, I hung up and called the Corderos. I explained we had to get there as soon as possible. We made a plan to leave in fifteen minutes. The hospital called back to tell me Elvis was not allowed in the room. If Dr. Welch was right, and Nick was going to die today, he was never going to get to see Elvis again. I started sobbing as I rushed into the bedroom to change out of my PJs. I rushed to get out of the house as fast as possible. Driving down Lookout Mountain on my way to the hospital, I spotted Anna walking up the hill with Elvis passed out in his baby carrier. I stopped and rolled the window down, trying to get the words out.

"Sister, I'm going to the hospital right now; I'm picking up the Corderos on the way. They told me Nick is dying. I have no idea when I'll be back!"

She looked as shocked and confused as I felt—she had the same déjà vu.

"I love you," she said. "Don't worry about Elvis."

When we got to the hospital, I was on the list but the Corderos weren't. Dr. Welch's message hadn't been communicated yet.

"Are you kidding me?!" I said.

At this point, everyone in the hospital knew who Nick was, who I was, who Nick's family was. They knew that we knew the rules; if we were all coming, it was because we had been approved. Yet every time, even up till the last day, they acted as if they had never seen me before when I arrived. Dr. Welch had told me every minute was critical, urged us to rush to the hospital, and now we were all waiting to be allowed upstairs. They finally allowed me to go up to his room but told the Corderos they had to go back outside and wait there while they checked the list. I ran up to Nick's room to find the nurses in the ICU; I was hoping they could intervene and get the Corderos through, too. The nurses started making calls, and I went into Nick's room to see him. His numbers were fine; he looked okay, and he seemed to be doing okay. I felt on the brink of losing it. I texted the Corderos with updates from my end, letting them know that Nick was okay. By the time they got up to Nick's room, they were furious; we all were. We'd been told that we should get here immediately, that Nick was dying. When we arrived, the Corderos were forced to wait outside on the street for an hour while they "checked the list," and now everything with Nick was apparently . . . normal?

We went into the meeting room with all the doctors, Debra, and, for the first time, a member of the hospital board's Ethics Committee. The Corderos and I were upset, confused, and exhausted as we sat there listening. The meetings always unfolded in the same order. They began with introductions, in case there was anyone new in the room, and then there was a review of everything that had happened thus far in Nick's case. We hated this part because hearing the saga that was our lives replayed each time was like a dagger stabbing us over and over. We were all trying to stay positive, but they were delivering the truth.

Nick was in a bad place again, they told us. Blood pressure medicines were back on, the vent settings were up, proning had helped initially, but it wasn't anymore. He was still in a state of acidosis, which meant the infection in his lungs wasn't improving. On top of all that, his mental status hadn't changed since he "woke up," and he wasn't showing any signs of getting off dialysis or moving his body. I sat there with my arms crossed, giving myself the hug I really needed as they spoke.

"It is getting to a point . . . we are not there yet"—Dr. Ng said—"but we're getting to a point where more harm is being done to Nick than help."

Dr. Welch sat there, nodding his head exaggeratedly, in agreement as Dr. Ng spoke.

"We have a couple options that we can talk about for Nick," he said. "The first we've mentioned before—comfort care. You aren't making any decision if you choose this—you are just allowing the machines to slowly be turned off so the body isn't assisted anymore. We would give Nick some morphine so he wouldn't feel any pain. He would drift off to sleep. At this point, that would probably happen within about thirty minutes once we stopped the machines."

Dr. Welch made more huge, exaggerated nods in agreement with this idea.

"The other option is that we keep moving forward as aggressively as possible, do bronch sweeps once a day to try to get rid of the secretions. We can continue to look into new treatments and trials to see if there is anything we are missing."

Dr. Welch began shaking his head left to right, as Dr. Ng offered this, signaling to us that this was *not* a good idea. His silent commentary was driving me crazy. I realized the Ethics guy was there to keep things in order and ensure that everyone abided by hospital rules and regulations. He was wearing a suit and had his notepad at the ready. He had not said a word thus far, but when Dr. Ng stopped talking, he finally asked me, "Amanda, how are you doing?"

Up until now, I had held it together in these meetings. I never overreacted, raised my voice, cried, or pointed fingers. All of those reactions, especially by this point, would have been entirely justifiable every step of the way. I had been on a roller coaster with this hospital for the last two months. I was fighting them every day to understand what was going on and to be allowed to see my husband. I was asked for my consent over and over again. I had three doctors who continually gave me different stories. I had sat in this meeting room and listened as I was told Nick was going to die—twice now. I was spending all my time and effort researching things to help him, just to have my ideas be immediately dismissed, to be told they weren't options. And, as the cherry on top, Dr. Welch told me that my husband's eyes were haunting him. *Him!* As if I were not being haunted by everything about this whole situation, every minute of every day.

Through all that—I kept it together. But today, after being called and told Nick was dying and to get here right away, and then having to fight with the reception staff and watch as the Corderos were told to wait outside on the street, and now to have to deal with Dr. Welch's personal game of charades while being presented with choices on the fate of my husband's life—it was the final straw, and I lost it.

"How am I?" I repeated. "I am—I think *we* are—utterly confused. I do not want to hurt Nick; that is the last thing I want to do, but I know he is fighting. You recommend comfort care? You say that *isn't* making a choice? But you also tell us that the minute you start taking machines away, he will die. So that is, in fact, making a choice to end my husband's life. I can't do that. I couldn't live with that decision, knowing that Nick is still fighting. And he *is* still fighting."

It was clear, immediately, that this was not the response they were expecting. But I was just getting started.

"This is not the first time you've told me, for sure, that he was going to die—soon! Not the first time that I've rushed here, said goodbye, sobbed, prayed, and made peace with losing him. When you allow me to be by his side—he fights and lives another day. How am I supposed to ignore that? You even agreed that he is a miracle; there was no other way to explain it! I know that Nick is sick, that he might not make it, but he is still fighting. I see that; we *all* see that. I had him tracking and smiling a week ago, a mere twelve hours after you said he had nothing left, no chance. He isn't giving up, so I am not going to give up!"

My voice rose and tears fell down my face. It was the first time I cried in a meeting, but I kept going.

"I am sick of being looked at like I'm crazy when I bring ideas to the table and having them instantly dismissed. I will never stop looking for something that can help him. I stay up for hours every night searching for something, anything, that might turn things around. And yes, some of the things are off the wall, but I don't care. I'm trying! You say Cedars is one of the most aggressive hospitals, willing to do things that other hospitals won't do. Why can't we try some new things? You keep saying that we are out of options, so what do we have to lose? We are running out of time! These new ideas *are* new options!"

The doctors looked stunned. They didn't say a word, and I continued my rant.

"I am exhausted from arguing over the visitation policies. I cannot play this guessing game with the hospital administration anymore. One day I'm allowed in; the next I'm not. One day I can come for two hours, the next day for four hours, the next day not at all. One day only

I'm allowed, the next day I should bring Elvis—wait, no, never mind—
he's not allowed! And then the next day we're all invited.

"You say you're worried about my emotional stability? Then please,
let me in this hospital to see him without these daily battles. I don't
even know who I'm fighting with! One day I'm told it's a board member
who won't let me in; the next day it's a head nurse or the ICU director.
I am sick of jumping through hoops. This is ridiculous, and I can't do it
anymore! You need to let Lesley in this hospital every single day as well
because she is his mother—and I need help here. I can't do this alone;
it's too hard. I am now a single mother. The minute I leave Nick to go
home to take care of Elvis, I feel terrible because I'm leaving Nick alone.
I'm being torn between being a mother and being a wife every day. I'm
no threat to this hospital. I don't go anywhere—I'm either here or at
home; I don't do anything but take care of Nick and take care of Elvis.
You can test me every day if you want to. I'll do whatever it takes.

"Today, we were called here, in a panic, on the premise that Nick
was about to die. We could barely breathe the whole way down here.
Then no one was on the list, and Nick's family had to sit outside on
the curb, for an hour! This was after Dr. Welch personally called and
told us to come immediately. He said that time was of the essence; noon
might be too late. This 'confusion' at the desk happens almost *every single day*. It's a daily, nonsensical battle for me to get in here to see my
husband, and I am sick of it.

"So you ask how I am doing . . . ? I'm not good! I'm sick of this uncertainty. I'm sick of being told that I should put him in comfort care.
I'm sick of being looked at like a sad puppy. I am strong, and Nick needs
help, and I am not giving up yet."

I took a huge breath when I finished, sat back in my chair, and wiped
the remaining tears away.

No one said a word for a while. The doctors and the Corderos had
never seen me react this way. It was the Ethics guy who spoke up first.

He apologized for the misunderstanding this morning, and every other day it had happened. He understood how this was causing extra stress and anxiety. He told me he would make sure that my getting into the hospital would no longer be an issue; he would make sure we could come every day without a problem. Dr. Ng chimed in next. He assured me that they would do anything and everything for Nick.

"Let's continue our course of aggressive care," he said. "There is no need to give up hope."

There was a moment of silence before Debra adjourned the meeting. I asked if the Corderos and I could stay in the room for a few minutes to talk. The hospital staff left the room. We all agreed that we didn't know if we were doing the right thing. We certainly didn't want to hurt Nick, but we couldn't give up yet either. Not just yet.

There was a knock at the door, and Dr. Ng walked in, barely a minute after he'd left.

My positive doctor came back to help. I think he hated how negative the meeting went and knew we all needed a bit of confidence before walking into Nick's room. He sat down and told us it was going to be okay. He promised he was going to do everything he could to get Nick better.

"He's forty-one; we fight," he said. "I have seen people survive with worse lungs than Nick's. We will keep doing daily bronchs and keep being aggressive. I'll talk to anyone you want me to, Amanda. I'm happy to look into anything you bring to the table."

He came back to give us a final cheer, which helped but also left us even more confused, as always. It was the blessing and curse of having several doctors with differing viewpoints and not knowing whose opinion to trust.

"I love Dr. Ng," Lesley said when he left.

"I know, Mom, I do, too," I said.

Meanwhile, the world outside the hospital got worse. Los Angeles was on fire as the protests grew more violent. There was already fear and anxiety in the air because of COVID, and now it was heightened as the world responded to George Floyd's murder. I had spent the last month seeing only the best of humanity, and this was a sad reality of injustice, violence, and hate. Driving to and from the hospital I saw the smoke, shattered windows, and damage done to the city from the riots. It was hard to believe this was my life and my city.

When I got home, I walked into the cabin to find my parents, Todd, and Anna waiting for me. I hadn't been able to call or update them since I'd left in a rush that morning. They had spent the day thinking, yet again, this was the end of the road. They were expecting me to walk in the door and say Nick was gone. I could tell they had all been crying, and I noticed for the first time how truly worn-out each of us looked—not just me. Everyone had red, puffy eyes; sunken faces; new worry lines. They tried to mask it when I walked in to be strong for me, but it was evident they had also spent the day in tears. I sank to the floor and sobbed as they huddled around me, wrapping their arms around me in a big family hug.

I didn't even know what to say anymore; I was out of words, emotions, and explanations. I had been up and down, again and again, since April 1, and it was now the end of May. I had said goodbye two times already; I had been certain it was the end. And I had watched a miracle happen, felt my hope that Nick would make it totally restored. Then my hope came crashing down again, and I was being told that keeping him alive was bordering on inhumane. I didn't know what to believe anymore, or whom to trust. But it felt like this was really the end. Nick had begun to look like someone who was dying, and every bit of me ached at the growing realization that I could lose him after all this. *Why would he have survived everything in the past two months only to die now?* That didn't make any sense to me. I told my family that night to please let everyone know that what I needed most right now was peace, quiet, and stillness. If Nick was going to pass, I didn't want flowers or other gifts delivered when he did. I didn't want people to call, text, ask how I was doing, or tell me they were sorry. I just needed silence.

Over the next two days, I picked up the Corderos and together we spent each day at the hospital, visiting in shifts. They would allow only two people in his room at a time—so we would take turns. They were the oddest days of all because I would sit in Nick's room, witnessing the trauma of the ICU, then look outside and hear the protests and watch tanks go by the hospital. It felt like I was in a movie about the end of the world.

I focused by praying for a miracle and keeping my faith that it would come. My sister, Traci, had called me at the hospital to give me some advice. "Amanda," she said, "sometimes we pray for a miracle, and God grants the miracle differently than we ask for."

These days at the hospital were long and tedious, trying to find comfort either standing by Nick's side or sitting in a waiting room. We were all in and out of sleep throughout the day and barely eating. On a break, Lesley and I went to sit outside for some fresh air and had a lovely heart-to-heart. She had lost her husband, Nick's father, only a few years before. So as my mother-in-law and a widow, she somehow was finding the strength to give me advice on how to get through the impossible—if losing Nick was to be our fate. She took my hand and, with tears in her eyes—both our eyes—assured me I'd be okay. She told me to fill my days with activities, to have a schedule, to keep busy. Have something to do each day. Try to make plans with friends.

"Elvis will help you a lot," she said, "because you'll have to take care of him, and smile for him."

She asked that we please stay in each other's lives and said how important it was for Elvis to know his Canadian family and roots.

"I wouldn't have it any other way, Mom," I said. "Of course he will; he always will."

"It'll be hard, though," she said, "especially if you find someone again one day—and you should, Amanda. I hope you know that I, we all, want you to live your life, and find love again. You're young, and you should find another man to love."

I was in awe of Lesley as she said this to me. Her firstborn son was dying, and here she was giving *me* a pep talk about dealing with grief and how she wants me to move forward, how it's okay for me to move on. It was so loving and selfless of her. It says everything about who she is.

I'll always remember that moment together, and that talk. It was beautiful and filled with great advice from a woman who had learned so much from her own pain and was strong enough to spend her lowest moment sharing her wisdom with someone else.

We walked back into Nick's room, and I asked for some time alone with him. I asked the nurse if I could climb into bed next to him; thankfully, she obliged my request. I needed him, and I hoped he needed me. I pulled a blanket over us and put on Alice Smith, an album Nick and I had loved to listen to when we started dating. The tears streamed down my face as I buried my head in my husband's frail chest as much as I could. It was thin and concave, and his collarbone stuck out sharply. I closed my eyes and hugged him close until I drifted off to sleep.

I woke up in a daze. I had passed out and didn't know for how long. I instantly felt terrible because it meant that the Corderos were all in the waiting room, unable to do anything. I got up and walked out to them, rubbing my eyes and apologizing for my nap. It had been two hours. They didn't even blink. They told me they were happy that I had had a good cuddle with him and a much-needed nap.

Dr. Welch found us all in the waiting room. He told us that he was going on vacation the following day, so he probably wouldn't see us again. He apologized for his frankness when providing his opinions, but he felt that he had to be honest with us. That's what he would want if he were Nick. He wanted us to know that he really cared for Nick and only hoped that he would make it. He wished us the best, and his manner was very heartfelt and sincere. I will admit that knowing he was gone was a small relief. His blunt honesty had been hard to deal with, and we really needed a high dose of positivity. Every doctor has a different style, and while Dr. Welch and I often didn't see eye to eye, I respected him. He was clearly a good doctor, and I appreciated his sincerity and all he did.

Before I went to bed that night, I reached out to my army on Instagram for help. My family had to move out of their current home in three days and we had found nothing else yet. I asked in a story that if anyone knew of a great rental that could accommodate eight people near Laurel Canyon to please reach out. I was never afraid to ask for help, especially now. When I started my business, I learned that people want to help; you just have to ask. It is impossible to do everything on your own. My motto became: "Ask for help. Ask for advice. It's a sign of strength, not weakness." Swallow your pride, put aside your fears—and ask. So I put my "ad" out to my army, hoping that someone might come to our rescue. Then I waited.

On the evening of May 30, my parents, Todd, and Anna were together at Brown Bear, getting ready for Sunday choir. The protests in LA had now become dangerous, and an eight p.m. curfew would go into effect that night. All the stores and restaurants were suddenly closing, and none of us had any food or groceries at home. The Corderos and I had spent the day at the hospital, but they kicked us out at seven thirty so we'd be home by curfew. By the time I got back to Brown Bear, Elvis was asleep already and Anna was jumping rope in the driveway. She stopped as I pulled in. I stepped out of the car and just collapsed onto the ground next to the front steps. It felt good to be out in the fresh air after being in the hospital room all day, and I was honestly too weak to stand. Anna sat down next to me and asked me how Nick was.

"He looks terrible, Annie," I confessed. "His numbers are awful: so, so low. He's lost every bit of color, and his face is sunken and so thin. He's lost fifty pounds now. He looks like someone who's about to die. I'll be shocked if he makes it through the night."

Anna put her arms around me. We just sat there on the concrete for a bit in silence, hugging. There was nothing to say.

I finally asked where everyone was.

"Todd, Diana, Mom, and Dad rushed home for curfew. We took all the food we had here to the Corderos', so they'd have something for dinner and breakfast. There wasn't much, but we gave them tons of wine!" she said.

"Oh, good," I replied. I was constantly worried about them. They were not familiar with LA, and I was always trying to ensure they were comfortable and fed, and felt like they were a part of our family.

"Do we have any food?" I asked her.

She flashed me a nervous smile. "Well, I tried to order things, but everything was closed. I'm hoping by some miracle the Meal Train is still coming. Since curfew is eight p.m., I thought it might get delivered, but so far nothing has come. It's not looking good."

I was starving; I hadn't left Nick's room to get lunch.

We sat in the driveway a little longer, just waiting to see if anyone was coming with food, but they weren't. It was time to admit defeat. Anna stood up and reached out her hand to help me off the ground. We walked together into the cabin with our arms interlaced. She told me to go shower, and she'd come up with something for us to eat. When I came out from the bathroom the table was set, and our meal was ready: Kraft instant macaroni and cheese, the sauce made with water because we had no milk. We had a side dish of leftover doughnuts from the day before and a bottle of Silver Oak Cabernet Sauvignon.

We sat down at the table, looked at our dinner, and then started laughing so hard tears came.

"This is, by far, the grossest meal I have ever had," I said.

"The grossest," she agreed, and we sat there hysterically laughing.

A few hours after Anna's ex-husband told her he wanted a divorce, she and I sat crying in a hug on the sidewalk at West Sixty-Ninth Street and Broadway. She had shrunk onto the ground the second she got out of the taxi she had taken from her apartment to mine. I threw on shoes and ran down to the street the second she called so that I could meet her outside. I could barely make out her words over the phone, but I knew something was wrong. A wave of sadness overtakes your entire body when someone you love is in pain. I had been through this exact type of pain—the precise moment of realizing your marriage, your world as you know it, is ending, and there is nothing you can do about it. We sat there on the sidewalk until she could stand up, then I held out a hand and we walked into my building together. She spent the next couple of days living with Nick and me. So I cleared my schedule to be with her and try to cheer her up. She had tickets to the musical *Frozen* for that week; she was supposed to be going with her husband. Anna loves Disney and saw *Frozen* in theaters more times than did most children I know.

"We are still going, sister," I told her when she asked what she should do with the tickets. "You and me! We'll make a whole day of it."

I decided to plan a day of fun and self-care before the show to keep Annie smiling.

I booked a morning yoga class for us, thinking it would be a good stress release for her and some nice meditation. As we flowed through poses, the teacher kept saying over and over again, "Take a deep breath, and then let it go!"

I noticed tears streaming down Anna's face. It was a therapeutic release and the perfect phrase for the moment. She had to let it go!

The instructor said it over, and over, and over again, "Let it go!"

Then it dawned on me—"Let It Go" was the hit song from *Frozen*!

"Sister," I whispered. "Let it go," I sang to the tune of the song.

She let out a laugh through her tears.

Our next stop on my agenda happened to be a cryotherapy session. "Oh my gosh," I said as we walked here, "cryotherapy is where you step into a freezing-cold chamber! This whole day is accidentally turning out to be *Frozen* themed!"

"Wow," she agreed, "it really is. First, 'Let It Go' and now we're going to freeze ourselves!"

It was her first time, and the cold is a bit shocking the first time you do it. I told her the key was to focus on something else and keep moving around and dancing while you're in there. When the three minutes started and the chamber suddenly filled with -230 degrees Fahrenheit air, she began to jump up and down, trying to keep warm. She yelled over the noise of the machine, "The cold never bothered me anyway!"

We started singing "Let It Go" together at the top of the lungs in the tiny room, laughing.

To continue the theme, we went to the show that night with our hair in elaborate braids. Anna weaved her long, blond hair into an Elsa-style side braid, and I wore my signature look: hair parted in the middle and a French braid on either side. "We even look the part," we giggled as we walked into the theater.

Nick's childhood friend from Toronto, Caissie Levy, was starring as Elsa, so after the show, we got to go to her dressing room and say hello. "I can't believe we get to go meet the *real* Elsa," Anna said. "This day is turning out to be fantastic."

We ended the night with one of our favorite things, also on theme: ice cream.

We walked from the theater to Serendipity on the Upper East Side, a kitschy café known for enormous, outrageous sundaes. One is more than enough for two people to share, but we each got our own and polished off every single bite.

As we walked home, Anna started crying as she thanked me for everything: for letting her stay with us, for making her smile, for the entire day of fun I had created to try to distract her from her pain. I had reminded her that there would be happy days ahead.

"Mands, this truly is a day themed around *Frozen*," she said while she hugged me, "because the moral of *Frozen* is that the most powerful kind of magic that exists . . . is the love between sisters."

sixteen

June 1 marked a new month, a shift in my mindset, and a different dynamic to our fight.

On May 1, I had written "Miracle May" on the whiteboard in Brown Bear. A month ago there had not been a shred of doubt in my mind that Nick would wake up, come off the ventilator, and have his Code Rocky. *He will be out of the ICU and in rehab by Elvis's birthday,* I told myself. *He will see his son turn one.*

May had not gone as planned, and my tune had changed considerably by the beginning of June, yet I was still hopeful. I still prayed every day and believed I would get a miracle, but Elvis's birthday was ten days away. I was coming to terms with the reality the doctors were discussing. In the very back of my mind, I had started to accept a world in which Nick would never make it to rehab.

But when I called the nurse the morning of June 1, Nick was doing better than he had in weeks. His settings were down, they took him off blood pressure medications, and he was alert and awake. This news shook me. It was another loop on the roller-coaster track. Two nights before, he'd looked like he was close to death. I was told it was inhumane to keep him alive. Now he was awake, improving, and looking good. This was the very reason I couldn't agree to move him into comfort care—things changed rapidly every day. Dr. Ng had given us goals for Nick's settings: numbers to watch for. Any time we neared them, we pointed out the good news immediately to the nurse on duty. We were clinging to every ounce of hope or good news and not trying to hide it. Our spirits rose when his numbers did, and we had a lot of things to celebrate.

June is the month of birthdays in our family. It begins with my sister Traci on the 2nd, then Hudson on the 3rd, Lesley on the 4th, Oliver on the 5th, my mom on the 8th, Elvis on the 10th, and then my niece, Eva, on the 13th. This year it was tough to be in any kind of "party mode," but since we are a family that celebrates the people we love in a big way, we decided we needed to make sure our month of birthdays went as normally as possible. We planned something fun for everyone; we wanted each person to have a special day, a cake, and a party.

As Elvis's birthday approached, I hoped that the hospital might allow me to bring him in to visit Nick so we could all be together, even if it was just for ten minutes. I knew my chances of that happening were low, but I had to try.

The Corderos and I were at the hospital all day during the first week of June.

Since curfew was still in place that week, we had to leave the hospital earlier, which felt awful. Every day the hospital was unsure of how long we would be able to stay for security reasons. We didn't want to leave Nick alone. He needed company. The irony did not escape me that, just when we had finally been told we could be at the hospital as much as we wanted, a curfew was established that limited our hours.

On June 3, we decided to celebrate Lesley's birthday in the hospital with Nick. It was very hard to tell what he was seeing, hearing, or comprehending. But it was Lesley's birthday, and before Amanda and Matt left to return to Canada, we needed to celebrate. We held Nick's hands and stood in a circle by his side as we sang to Lesley and wished her the best day possible. None of us were sure what that meant right now or how "happy" we could be, but we did it anyway. Lesley put on such a brave face through this and shed just a few tears. Her courage astounded me. Despite how hard it was for us, I'm glad we had this "party"—because I know Nick would have wanted us to. If he could comprehend what was going on, I knew he would love that he was with his family for his mom's birthday and that we were celebrating. Matt and Amanda had to say their goodbyes that day, so they each took ample alone time with their brother, knowing it might be the last time they ever saw him. I couldn't imagine what they were feeling. I had spent the first two months of this battle just thinking as his wife. Now, being in the hospital with the Corderos made me think: What if that was my brother? What if that was my sister? What if that was my son?

As they each walked out of his room that day, in tears, we were all silent. They had lives and families of their own they had to return to. No one knew what was going to happen to Nick, how long he had to live. He could pass away that evening or be in the ICU in this exact state for another six months. They couldn't stay here forever, so they had to make the very difficult choice to say goodbye and hope they would get to see their brother again.

Later that night, we had another party for Lesley with my family to celebrate with her and say goodbye to Amanda and Matt. My family was getting to know Lesley so well, and I knew that would make Nick happy. Our two families hadn't spent much together because they lived in different countries. Now we had had time to sit around and share stories and really bond. With Amanda and Matt leaving, we told Lesley that our house was her house now. She was family, and we wanted to see her every day that she wanted to see us.

Anna continued to be on primary Elvis duty since we were still living in Brown Bear. He was warming up to everyone, but not quite at the point yet of letting other people hold him. She put aside everything else to make Elvis her priority out of pure love, not obligation. I couldn't believe how she had stepped up and completely learned how to be a substitute mom. I teased her that this was probably making her rethink having children, but she said that, thanks to Elvis, she now was more sure then ever that she wanted a baby one day. I knew once we could all move in together, it would be easier for her. Thankfully, my plea for help in finding a more permanent house was answered later that week.

We got an email from the wife of a celebrity who had been following the whole story. She saw my family was looking for a home and wanted to help. In her email she wrote that she knew what it was like to go through a medical trauma. Her husband had been diagnosed with cancer a few years before. There was a five-bedroom house in Laurel Canyon with a pool, hot tub, and giant front yard that she offered to us for as long as we needed it. She wasn't going to charge us a dime; in fact, she wanted to also cover our groceries and any other expenses that our family had. I didn't know what to say. How do you accept that kind of generosity? How do you even begin to thank someone for it?

When I told my parents, my dad was stunned. "Amanda," he said, "I have prayed for that man every morning since the day he announced he had cancer. There has never been a day I didn't ask God to help him and his family."

I had chills. It felt like a gift sent right from heaven, an answer to prayers.

The house was like our own personal resort. There were four bedrooms downstairs and an upstairs area where the kids could stay. There was a closed-off dining room that Todd and Diana could use as an office as they tried to work. There was a huge kitchen and living room where we could spend time as a family and Elvis could crawl around. But the most incredible thing was the view. The house was high up on a hill on Crescent Drive, just off Mulholland. It had a panoramic view over Los Angeles that looked like something straight out of a movie. There was an outdoor table for ten, pool loungers, and umbrellas.

When one of my friends saw it, she said, "Amanda, a lot of your life sucks right now. But this bit—this is *good!*"

We graciously accepted the generous offer, and Anna and I decided to leave Brown Bear and move in with the rest of the family at the end of that week. Everyone helped as we moved out. I had foolishly thought it would be quick and easy, but I had completely underestimated the amount of stuff we had accumulated in the last few months. Everything had to be sorted: what we actually needed at the new Laurel Canyon house, what we needed to take to the family house, and what could be donated. Elvis and I had tons of things to go through, but the most difficult was Nick's things: guitars, amps, vinyl, books, toiletries, and his entire closetful of clothes. I had no idea what to do with it all.

I knew that even if he left the hospital, he would be living in rehab for the next year, at least. He had lost almost sixty pounds now; none of these clothes were going to fit him anymore. I decided to make a call and packed it all up to be donated, except for a few things I knew Nick really loved and a few things I wanted for myself, as a way of keeping him close.

It was difficult to leave the place that had been our first "LA home" in a way, but it also felt good to be out. It was now full of so many sad memories; moving out felt like a fresh start. Now, Anna and I could wake up every morning and be with the family right away; we could spend time outside and in the pool. We moved into the master bedroom together since we were already roommates, and I didn't want to be alone. We turned the enormous walk-in closet into Elvis's nursery, so he finally had his own room and we could actually get some sleep at night.

Though we lived there for only two months, this house became our home. We spent all day there, swimming in the pool, playing with the kids in the yard, and grilling outside. We had family meals around the table, workouts on the terrace, and long chats in the living room. At night, the view was like a scene from La-La Land, the city of stars shining just for us. In between the nightly birthday celebrations that first week, I did shifts with Lesley in the hospital.

We were back in a pattern of no changes: nothing getting worse, but nothing getting better. I did trust Dr. Ng was doing what was best for Nick. He came into the room to check on him continuously and was always happy and available to answer any of our questions.

"What is our biggest obstacle right now; what is Nick's biggest problem that needs to be solved?" I asked him one day.

"He can't release carbon dioxide from his lungs," he said.

He left Nick's room, and I went to my Instagram army. I posted another "ad" on my story, asking for anyone who had help or insight into this specific problem. Within minutes I had suggestions in my inbox, and they just kept coming. I sat in Nick's room writing everything down on a napkin, a list of ten people to contact. I had a fire in my belly; there were a lot of exciting things that people were suggesting that I hadn't heard of.

One cryptic message from someone I didn't know said only, "You need to call a woman in Brooklyn named Alice." I wrote the number down on the top of my list and was about to call when Dr. Ng walked into the room.

There were bits of paper everywhere with scribbles. Nick's room had become my medical research office.

"So I leave for thirty minutes, and you've got a full investigation going on?" he said.

"Dr. Ng," I joked, "when this is over, you're going to want to hire me—but you won't be able to afford me!"

I went down my list, spouting off some of my findings to him. Some things couldn't be done. Some weren't applicable because of Nick's status or condition. Some seemed possible, but Dr. Ng would need to do more research. Some I knew wouldn't be right, but I asked anyway because we had nothing to lose.

"Keep going," he said. I promised him I'd have more questions and ideas for him on his return.

"I don't doubt it, Amanda," he said.

I still had half a dozen people to call, and the first one was Alice.

I didn't know her; I hadn't ever talked to her or heard of her or her family, but she picked up the phone and greeted me like we had been friends for years.

"Amanda," she said in a deep, raspy voice, with a thick Brooklyn accent. "Amanda, I want to help you. My husband, he had COVID. He just got home, and he's still recovering. My best friend, Susie, has it now. We have to stop this virus, Amanda. We have to find a cure. I am trying to help people, and my friend saw your post on Instagram and told me I have to talk to you."

I loved her already.

Alice told me that she was familiar with who I was, but not because of this story. She said that years ago I had taught a fitness class at the Jewish Community Center in Brooklyn. She hadn't been able to attend but heard about it afterward. When her friend told her about my story, she remembered who I was and wanted to help. I remembered this class and how I almost had to turn it down. It wasn't easy to get there from Manhattan, and at the time, I was already teaching six or seven classes a day. It was a trek to get out there, particularly during a New York winter. But I ended up accepting the offer because I was inspired by a whole group of women who wanted to dance and work out together. I remember being so glad afterward that I had gone. It shows how things you do in life sometimes make an impact without your realizing it, and that any moment can lead to something significant years later. Because I had helped them, this kind woman was doing everything in her power to help me now, and it sounded as if she had a lot of power.

Alice and her husband were benefactors, both incredibly giving in times of need, especially to hospitals. I dove into telling her Nick's story, every single detail of what had happened from day one until where we were today. They put me in touch with their good friend Jeff, who called me a short time later to tell me he would reach out to Cedars on my behalf. He was also going to assemble the best team for Nick, with doctors from around the country, and check on me to make sure Nick and I were okay. I didn't know how to react, other than to say "Thank you!" repeatedly. The whole call had felt like a scene from a movie.

"We want you to call us every day. We want to know his numbers every day. Let's stay in touch. The only way to get through this and save our people is by sharing information," Alice said.

I couldn't have agreed more.

That same day, I received a direct message from one of my Broadway friends who said I had to call someone named Dr. Larry. He knew Nick because he supported the theater where *A Bronx Tale* did their out-of-town tryout before coming to Broadway. We clicked the second I called him, and we spoke that day and then every single day until Nick passed away.

"I want to help," he began. "What I do is help people through these situations. I can be a sounding board between the hospital and you. I'm happy to give you my opinion, talk to Nick's doctors, and call anyone you need me to. Whatever you need, I'm here."

We started talking about Nick's case right away, and I loved hearing his ideas and knowing that I had more support from yet another doctor, especially one who already knew Nick. I thought back on the last hour, realized how much new help I had, and was overwhelmed with gratitude.

I left Lesley at the hospital for an hour and went to have an Elvis break and see my parents. I couldn't wait to tell them all this new news. I was on a high, filled with energy and hope. I recounted the day's events as if I were doing a one-woman show on Broadway. I had all my family on the patio listening to every word I said. So much information and help had flooded in. It really felt like this new team that had assembled— Alice, her friend Jeff, and Dr. Larry—were here to save the day. It was as if New York City was coming to my rescue.

On the way back to the hospital, I got a call from the head doctor at Cedars-Sinai, Dr. Paul Noble. He had just gotten off the phone with Jeff and had then called to ask, "What do you need? What can I do?" I couldn't believe I was speaking to the top-ranking doctor at Cedars-Sinai! I wasn't going to let this go to waste. I rattled off a list of things I wanted to be done and checked for Nick, and the doctor said he would get right on it and would get back in touch with me when he had information and answers.

All of this just because I asked for help, I thought.

"God is good! Thank you, God," I prayed.

I often think about all the help I received. I think of all the unlikely connections, the total strangers, and the friends in high places who rushed to my aid. It was because of them that I was allowed in the hospital with Nick, that my family had a beautiful home to stay in, that the Corderos had been allowed into the country while the borders were closed. I thought about everyone who was suffering, who would suffer in the months to come and did not have the same team, army, and friends with the power to help them move mountains. I never let it escape me that while I was in a terrible situation, I was also quite fortunate.

With everything else happening, I was still in the middle of our home renovation.

Todd had become my house coordinator by this point, and I had given my contractor, Bill, and my designer, Michelle, carte blanche to do whatever they thought was best. I told all of them, "I trust you." I had never owned, renovated, or designed a home, and I was too busy to worry about it. They took over and worked tirelessly, with the goal of having the house done by August.

When my mom's birthday came, we decided to go back to my friend's house on the beach in Malibu to celebrate. My mom is the one who taught us to celebrate one another and started the tradition of going all out for our birthdays. We wanted to make sure she had a special one. So we packed up a cooler with sandwiches and rosé, and drove toward the beach. It was a gorgeous day, and within seconds of getting to the house, Todd's children, Oliver and Hudson, had stripped down to their underwear and were running toward the ocean. It felt so special to be in the sunshine, by the water, and feel the sand under our toes. Going to the beach had been a simple thing before COVID; now it was an enormous privilege. We all ran down to the shore like kids, and it was a rare, joyous moment that month when life felt normal.

Elvis was up next. I couldn't believe he was turning one. I had not planned on throwing him a big party, but after Jennifer Love Hewitt had so kindly offered her help, Anna was working with companies she had put us in touch with—including Los Angeles's premier party planner, balloon specialist, and bakery—to throw Elvis a first birthday party more elaborate than my best one had been. The morning of his birthday there was a giant balloon wall that said ELVIS and picnic tables with decorative records, candy-colored Mustangs, and confetti. There were mini-doughnuts made into vinyls, cake pops that looked like microphones, and Rice Krispies treats with photos of Elvis dancing on them.

I had ordered 1950s glasses, scarves, and saddle shoes for my mom, Anna, and me. We got dressed up in our theme first thing in the morning and did a music class on Zoom, thanks to all of Elvis's baby "friends" from before COVID. Elvis sat on my lap while I bounced him on my knees, and we sang "Three Little Birds." He was smiling ear to ear; he had always loved his music class.

Lesley took the morning shift at the hospital so I could be with Elvis, but we FaceTimed with Nick right when we woke up. Luckily, it felt so busy at the house with everything being prepped that it kept me distracted from what I thought would be an extremely hard day.

Our driveway at the house was a massive horseshoe, so we set up outside with 1950s tunes blasting and greeted all of our friends from far away as they drove through our drive-by birthday parade. Elvis's Stroller Buddies arrived in full costume; they had gotten the memo on the theme and show people never miss an opportunity to come in costume. Everyone who came to the parade arrived with gifts and balloons, and there was much singing and dancing. I felt so blessed.

I headed to Cedars after the last car left. I'd planned a little slide show for Nick: pictures of Elvis from the day he was born. I also had videos recorded from that morning's activities. I brought with me cards that people had sent to Elvis so I could read them to Nick. I wanted to keep things as cheery as possible for him today. Back at home, the official party started, made up of family and close friends. My dad grilled hot dogs, and we all sat in the backyard in the sunshine. I couldn't believe Elvis was one. He had grown into such a sweet, loving, curious baby boy. Nick would be so proud.

W hile I was still pregnant, I ordered a baby book for Elvis. I wanted it early so that I could get a head start on filling things out. The first page of the book had a question for both parents to answer, "What do you wish for your baby?"

I wrote, "Today is one month before your due date. We can't wait for you to arrive! Be a dreamer, be confident, be strong, be wise, love everyone, have compassion, go for your dreams, have faith, show humility, be kind, and work hard!"

Nick wrote, "Your Mom said it all. I hope you're kind, confident, and happy. I hope you find joy and that you're able to see the wonder in the world. I hope you know above all that you are loved."

I always get asked why my family is so close, how we love each other so much and have such a tight bond. It's something my siblings and I have often talked about as we got older and started having families of our own. We have searched for an exact formula, or thing to pinpoint, but that one thing doesn't exist. We have come to agree that it was the example our mom and dad set with their own lives, the lessons they taught us, and the things they gave us that cannot be bought: unwavering faith in God, unconditional love, encouragement, support, honesty, and joy. My parents never pushed us in any direction with school or passion, and they never missed a show or recital once we decided our paths. They were strict with us with rules, manners, and chores, so we never took anything for granted. They gave us all space to make our own choices and mistakes, but they were right there to help when we failed. We watched my dad work so hard, every day of the week, to provide for us. We watched my mom be completely selfless and devote her entire life to her family. We witnessed their love and commitment to each other, and we were continuously shown how much they loved each one of us.

On the morning of his first birthday, I wrote Elvis another letter:

Dear Elvis,

Happy 1st birthday, my amazing baby boy! You are the light of my life! I woke up today with you in my arms, cuddled up next to me, and I was reflecting on a year ago this morning. What that was like, and where we were. You came and made us a family, and I know your Daddy would have loved to be here today. He misses

you, Elvis, I can tell when I visit him. It's day 70 in the ICU for him,
and I know he's fighting for you.

   We love you so much.

      Love,

      Mommy

I didn't let myself think about how heartbroken I was that day. Instead, I just masked it with a smile and focused on all the joy Elvis
brought me. It was devastating that Nick was not there, but as I looked
around me, I couldn't help but feel very blessed. I saw my parents, Lesley, Todd and his family, Anna, and my best friends there to celebrate.
If it were normal times, I knew they wouldn't all have been able to be
here. That was a gift. Throughout the party, I often wanted to cry, but
there was my beautiful little boy, sitting on his own in a chair, his
face, hands, and shirt completely covered in chocolate as he inhaled a
miniature, record-shaped doughnut. He was smiling ear to ear, and so
I was, too.

seventeen

I was in the hospital with Nick when Elvis took his first steps. He had already been pulling himself up to a standing position and then balancing there for the last week, so we knew the steps were coming. It happened one afternoon when my mom and Lesley were sitting on the floor chatting while Elvis played. They said, "All of sudden, he just walked by!"

They told me they held their breath as they counted ten steps, then twenty.

I felt my heart drop when I first heard I missed it, realized Nick missed it. Neither of us should have missed that milestone. But it was special that both of his grandmas got to be there for it. I had been there, and would be there, for so many significant firsts. I was happy they had this one. I immediately kissed him when I got back from the hospital that day and congratulated him.

"Okay, Elvis," I said, putting him down and walking a few steps back, "walk to Mama!"

Seven steps later, Elvis was back in my arms and grinning with pride.

He stumbled around from that point, trying to keep his balance, and he walked with one arm out like a baby Superman. With him now walking around the house, containing him became a little more complicated.

He could get into things we hadn't even realized were potential trouble. I found him trying to pull discarded pizza out of the trash can one morning!

Nick's day-to-day at the hospital became extremely hard on us. We were battling his infections and blood pressure medicines. One day he would be great; the next morning he was horrible. I started calling it the ICU dance and began to feel numb to the situation. I could no longer let my hopes rise and fall with his numbers. I was approaching eighty days of this, and I think everything I had been through was taking a severe toll—I had become almost emotionless at times.

I wasn't the only one feeling burned out. Lesley and my parents were exhausted. My siblings had been doing this since April, too. A week after Elvis's birthday, Todd left to go back to San Francisco for some time alone in his own house, to just enjoy the quiet and clear his mind. Anna rented a car and did a short road trip to Joshua Tree for the same reason. Having them gone for a few days was a little reality check for me: this bubble wouldn't last forever; I wouldn't always have my family living with me to distract me and help make everything more manageable.

Nick wasn't making any measurable progress. They had started Exosome therapy on June 3; hoping the cells would help to regrow tissue.

I was ecstatic that they were finally trying something new. But after a few days we could tell the stem cells weren't helping as much as we had hoped. The only benefit we saw was his white blood cell count was going down, which indicated this infection was getting better. Meanwhile, new infections seemed to pop up every other day. He would lie quiet and motionless for hours while I visited, and then all of a sudden, he would look up at me and answer questions by moving his eyes. These moments restored our hope, but they were rare and fleeting. Sitting there one day, I thought of one of my favorite Bible verses, Ephesians 6:10. It's about dressing yourself in "the armor of God" so that you can walk through the most challenging times feeling strong. I needed armor; I needed to have thick skin. I needed my faith.

I was so thankful to have Lesley there, not only to help take care of Nick but to have someone else who understood the toll the visits took, and the complexity of emotions you feel when you're in this sort of situation. I was also grateful that I wasn't alone in making decisions, hearing updates, and tracking numbers. The roles of mother and wife are so different, and Nick now had those two very different types of love and support every day.

Lesley also chatted often with the nurses, as did I. We loved hearing about them. They were incredibly smart and hardworking; Nick would have the same nurse in his room for three or four days, so we got to know them quite well.

The next morning, my in-box flooded with links to an article about a COVID patient in Chicago who had successfully received a double lung transplant. Thanks to Dr. John, within an hour I was on the phone with the surgeon who had done it. This idea, which had once terrified me, now was exhilarating: a new hope for something that could save Nick. So I dove in and started mapping out all the details. I learned that I'd have to hire a medical jet to transport Nick to Chicago—but thankfully the GoFundMe would allow me to do that, if need be. I'd have to sell our house and relocate across the country. We'd have to live in Chicago for a few years while he got strong enough for the surgery, recovered, and did rehab. *Whatever it takes*, I thought.

I was pumped on adrenaline. This was our Hail Mary pass, our last shot. Dr. Ng and I talked to the transplant doctor at Cedars the next day to see if this was a possibility, and he shed more light on the situation. To even become a candidate, there are specific criteria that you have to meet. You have to be able to sit up and stand up. You need to be able to move your arms and legs. You cannot be on dialysis or blood pressure medications. Currently, all Nick could do was move his eyeballs up, down, left, and right. Standing up seemed light-years away. I kept faith, since I knew nothing was going to work overnight. I had been told from the beginning—this is a marathon, not a sprint. But time was not on our side. Every day that passed, Nick was becoming weaker, more dependent on the machine. Every day, his lungs were becoming more damaged. He needed the transplant to walk, but he needed to walk in order to qualify for the transplant.

There were so many things that were dependent on something else. He needed to make progress to get better, but he couldn't make progress because he was always on and off the medications that were either preventing progress or causing new problems. Dr. Ng had been doing bronchial sweeps almost every other day to keep Nick's lungs clear. Some days the results from that sweep were great; other days, we were back to copious secretions and even flaking skin from his esophagus. I got brave and started watching the bronch sweeps to learn and see for myself what we were dealing with. It was terrifying to watch. I prayed every day for some kind of good news, some small change that would give us hope. At this point, even the smallest action would have been a huge step in the right direction. If he could blink, close his jaw, move a finger, even cough—it would have been game-changing.

The doctors hadn't brought up comfort care again since the meeting in which I'd lost it. Lesley and I hadn't discussed it either. If Nick's eyes were open and moving, it was not something we were willing to consider. It is an impossible task to try to decide what someone wants when he cannot speak. But Nick was fighting, every day, and to us, that meant he was making the decision to live. As long as he was fighting, we were going to fight, too.

When Father's Day came, I found myself aching inside as I watched everyone celebrate and read people's lovely dedications to their dads on Instagram and Facebook. I couldn't help but feel it was unfair, and I wondered what life would be like for Elvis without his dad if Nick did not survive. I asked myself all day, *Why did this happen to Nick?* He deserved to be home, healthy, and celebrated. Nick had wanted to be a father so badly; he had told me many times how he knew at ten years old that he wanted to be a dad. But he had always wanted a little girl, and he had planned to name her Ava.

M y sister Traci gave us instructions before we went to our first ultrasound, where we would get to hear our baby's heartbeat. She said, "Make sure they tell you the number of the heartbeat; a high number is usually a girl, and a lower number means a boy."

As we heard our baby's heartbeat for the first time, our own hearts exploded. It was 165, a high number, and even the nurse confirmed this old wives' tale is usually a good indicator. Nick was ecstatic. Little Ava was a step closer to reality. On Thanksgiving that year, we flew to Ohio to be with my family and do a gender-reveal ceremony. We had gotten the result a week before but sent it right to Anna without looking at it ourselves. She had planned a game for us to play with a dozen eggs that would reveal the baby's gender. You take a dozen eggs, boil all but one of them, and color half blue and half pink. The raw egg is pink if it's a girl or blue if it's a boy. Each parent-to-be then takes a different color egg and, simultaneously, hits the eggs against their foreheads. When the raw egg breaks, that egg's color reveals the gender. We got all the way through the eggs and were down to the last two! On the count of three, we each cracked an egg against our foreheads. Mine broke, yolk running down everywhere as the tears came, too. It was blue; we were having a boy! Nick went into shock.

"A boy," he said. "A boy? We're having a boy?"

He wasn't prepared.

After the shock wore off, we started thinking of names as a family.

I had been entirely on board with Ava, but nothing for a boy was really sticking for me. I kept testing names by saying my name and then the suggested baby name to see if I liked it . . .

Amanda and Axel.

Amanda and Leo.

Amanda and Raphael.

I didn't like any of them. I suggested going through musicians we love, since music was such a part of Nick's life, and Elvis came to my mind immediately.

Amanda and Elvis.

I loved it right away.

"No," Nick said. "No way! Everyone will think I named him Elvis because I love Elvis's music. It will be the first question we're asked every time we introduce him to people. 'Oh, you guys must be huge Elvis Presley fans.'"

I shook my head in protest. "No, they will not, and even if they do, who cares? Once people know our little guy as Elvis, it will be *his* name. I really like it. Amanda and Elvis. Amanda, Nick, and Elvis."

For nine months, we fought about the name. I kept telling Nick to bring his ideas to the table, and I would happily consider them. But he only had one name he liked for a boy—Eddie. His dad's name was Eduardo, and he liked the idea of naming our son after him. I liked the idea, too; I just felt that Eddie was too common a name for us. Nick would continuously test the names out on friends to gauge their reaction. Every time he said, "Amanda wants to name our kid Elvis," people would respond, "Whoa, that's cool. I like it!" I would smirk, and Nick would shake his head. He had hoped they would side with him. He didn't give up this routine right up to a month before the birth, on our babymoon in Grand Cayman. I heard him deliver his line to a complete stranger in the pool. "She wants to name our baby Elvis."

"Oh my gosh, our daughter's name is Presley!" she exclaimed. "Elvis! That's so cool. You never hear that."

Not too long afterward, after nine months of arguing, he conceded, admitting he "sort of knew" all along it was the perfect name for him, but he just had to fight it. I felt my blood boil, but I shut up because I had won. We would soon be Amanda, Nick, and Elvis.

After fifty-six hours of labor, the nurse asked for the baby's name.

"Elvis," I said proudly.

She turned straight around to look us in the eye.

"Elvis? Wow, I have been in this hospital for thirty years, and I have never written down that name before. It's so cool," she said.

Nick looked at her with a proud smile and said, "I know, right?"

I had asked to bring Elvis to the hospital on Father's Day, but the answer was no. I visited Nick in the morning and found him more alert and aware than I had in days. His numbers were great, all things considered, and I played him videos of Elvis walking. His eyes connected with the screen as I showed him, and he followed Elvis as he moved around. I knew how badly he must have wanted to say something. I would have loved to hear his voice, know what he was thinking. But he couldn't, and it broke my heart. We FaceTimed with many friends that day from the hospital, so people could wish him a happy Father's Day. Then we spent the rest of the day as a family, celebrating my brother and my dad. I focused on how lucky I was to have them there instead of how much I hurt inside. My little boy was without his dad today, but he did have his grandpa and uncle, and they loved him just as much as a father would.

With visits monotonous, the hospital drama finally over, and my massive support network now fully trained and adjusted to life here, everything became relatively calm and routine for a while. It was very hard to have only three hours in the hospital each day. I went there like I was going to work. I did the same drive, passed the same people at the reception desk, and went directly to Nick's room, which was now my office. I said a prayer as soon as I got there, gave him pep talks and speeches, and said another prayer at the end of my visit. I sang him "Our House" every day just before I departed. I wanted to leave him on this happy note; it was one of his favorite songs, and I told him to visualize the two of us sitting at our home, drinking wine on the patio, looking at each other like, *Wow! We did this. We made it. We got through this.*

Some days he was alert, focused, and aware. And others, it was like he wasn't in there at all. It was hard to leave him in either state. If he was just lying there, lifeless, I felt guilty and sad leaving him there alone. But if he was alert, I felt almost worse leaving. He could see me go if he was awake. I couldn't imagine what he thought as he saw me walk out the door. I always walked to my car, feeling defeated, and had to adjust my mindset on the drive home.

Thankfully, though, the house had become such a happy place, and we had a nice routine. We spent the afternoons swimming in the pool, walking through the Canyon, and running errands for the house. Lesley came to the house as soon as her shift was done, and by seven each night, we were all together and ready for dinner. We sat around the table, and Lesley and I shared updates with each other from our respective shifts, filling the family in on what the doctors had said that day and how Nick looked. Anna helped me get Elvis ready for bed, and then we returned to the kitchen for dessert and to watch the sunset. We had a spectacular view from the house, as the sun slowly sank into the Hollywood Hills each night. It fell perfectly between the tall cypress trees and reminded us how beautiful the world is. We sat around the table for hours at night, just talking. Aside from the overarching sadness of our reality, it felt like we were on a family vacation: we were together in a beautiful home, with perfect weather, good food, and wine. It saved me in many ways, but it also hurt me so much knowing how Nick would have cherished these times.

In late May, the governor of California began lifting restrictions that had been in place with the Safer at Home order, and it became public knowledge that hospitals were able to resume a more normal visitation policy. My army was ecstatic. In everyone's mind, this would be the first time I was allowed to visit. I couldn't tell the truth, that I had been visiting all along, but I also couldn't fake the emotions and story of seeing him for the first time. So I got on Instagram and expressed how happy I was to see him, leaving out any kind of language like "for the first time." I shared a picture of his hand in my mine, cropping out his forearm so you couldn't tell how skinny it had become.

I took a photo of Nick to send to the family, and it shocked even me. I saw him every day, yet in the photo it was undeniably apparent just how much weight he had lost, how thin he had become. He looked like half of himself, a shell of his former body. Nick was also suffering from bedsores by this point; the largest one, on his tailbone, was getting worse by the day. The nurses were turning him every two hours to try to help it and changed the dressing frequently to keep it clean. We could not let him develop any more infections. One day the plastics team came to check on this bedsore and see how deep it had become. I was in the room, so I had the option of staying while they examined it. As they pulled the blankets off Nick and turned his body onto its side, I almost fainted. His amputated leg had no muscle tone and just flopped over to the side. His bones were protruding out of his skin. I hadn't seen Nick's whole body since he had been admitted to the hospital, and I was in shock. The bedsore was huge; it must hurt him. I almost had to look away, but I forced myself to watch and listen to the doctors and learn. I had been briefed on this; it was something that they had talked to us about; I just realized that day, though, how serious it was. For Nick to be a lung transplant candidate, this, too, would have to be healed, or at least almost healed.

"How can it heal, though, if he continues to lie in bed? Isn't the only way to heal it by moving around, sitting up, walking?" I asked.

I don't know why I even asked this question. I knew the answer was yes.

In some ways, the eighty days that had passed felt like a lifetime, but in retrospect, it had been only eighty days. That's a short time for such a drastic change. Not even three months ago, my life had been completely normal. Nick had been a healthy, six-foot-five, 225-pound man. Now I sat beside his hospital bed, and it was hard to recognize any trace of him. He weighed 148 pounds. His face was half the width it had been; his eyes looked enormous and were always covered in Vaseline to keep them hydrated while they were open since he couldn't close his eyelids all the way. His eyelashes had grown long and were also thick with the same jelly. His hair was greasy, slicked back, and longer than ever, and the hospital staff was grooming his facial hair, so his mustache and beard looked pretty odd. They were nurses, not barbers. His jaw was always hanging open; he couldn't close it on his own, even though I worked tirelessly with him on the physical therapy exercises when I was there. The PT team had shown me a series of exercises to help strengthen his jaw muscles, and though they helped a little, his jaw was always at least half open, showing his teeth, which now were covered in a film and looked exaggerated against his thin neck and protruding cheekbones. I brought tweezers and scissors one day and groomed his eyebrows when the nurse wasn't in the room. I wasn't sure I was allowed to, but I wanted to help him look as normal as possible. Because of the blood pressure medications, his hands and toes were still swollen, ballooned to twice their normal size, and his skin was leathery, like he was wearing a set of thick work gloves. Most of his fingertips and the toes on his left foot were still black; one day they're going to fall off completely, the doctors told me. In the best-case scenario, he would have two fingers on his right hand and no toes on his left foot.

During my visits, I was still giving Nick big speeches and encouraging him to be optimistic. Dr. Ng told me the other doctors on the floor had observed my behavior and asked him, "Does Amanda know? Does she understand how critical her husband is? How serious this is? She's in here smiling and singing . . . Does she not get it?"

Dr. Ng always had my back. He replied, "What do you want her to do? Mope around and be sad?"

I knew everything. I knew how bad it was. How increasingly slim his chances were. But I also knew focusing on that wasn't going to help me and wasn't going to help him. I was preparing myself the whole time that I might lose him, but I had him right now. He was still alive and fighting. Why should I let my mind go to that dark place when, instead, I could sit here and pray? I could sing, smile, and believe. The doctors on the floor were worried about my mental status, but I was only worried about Nick.

"Nick," I told him, "you can't let your mind get lost. You have to focus.

"Focus on a vision, a dream. You're standing on a stage, at a sold-out concert! You are playing 'Live Your Life,' and Elvis and I are in the wings, and we're cheering you on, and I'm pregnant again, and we're doing this! That will be your life, Nick; that will be our life."

"Don't get lost; get focused" became my refrain that week. If he believed that he could do this, then his body would respond—I hoped.

E very January, I start the year by making a vision board. It's not flashy or fancy. I find a cheap poster board, grab a stack of old magazines, and, armed with a pair of scissors, start cutting out whatever speaks to me. Sometimes it's letters I piece together to form words, sometimes it's images, sometimes it's people I admire or dream of working with. Every year it's different, and I hang the finished product in my bedroom. As the months go by, I find that these things I put on the board slowly come to fruition. It's not always the way I planned or when I planned, but they happen.

In 2020, as I prepared to do my vision board, I got Nick one, too, and told him he had to participate. But he wasn't into it. As I combed through page after page, snipping and tearing and finding things I wanted to add, Nick slowly flipped through his magazine, looking bored. When he grabbed for the scissors, finally settling on something, I was eager to see what it was. For the next thirty minutes, while I cut out at least one hundred things for my own board, Nick sat at the end of the table, meticulously cutting out an enormous picture of RuPaul. I was puzzled, and when I asked him why RuPaul, he answered bluntly, "Because she's amazing."

An hour later, he had made just two other additions to his board. The Geico gecko, and a picture of Diane Warren, a songwriter whom he admired. It was his vision board, not mine, but I couldn't help but be skeptical of his choices.

I hung my board up as I always do, and Nick put his in a drawer. I had forgotten all about it. When I pulled it out one day, I realized that, because the board had been stashed in a drawer, with things piled on top of it, the board had been damaged. A tear went through the paper, and RuPaul's right leg had been torn almost halfway off. I just stared at it. After flipping through stacks of magazines, Nick had chosen this image: RuPaul—an actor, singer, songwriter, and television personality. She embodied transformation, success, and living your life—everything Nick was going through.

The only other notable thing on his board was the gecko—so I googled its meaning. The first thing that came up said this: "Geckos symbolize that there is always hope for rebuilding our own lives." They represent rebirth and life cycles and are the symbol of good luck in a home. I was speechless. I instantly shared the story on Instagram, and then I studied my own board that evening, noting the images and words I had chosen to clip out and paste onto the board.

Bestselling author, a check I wrote out to myself for a million dollars, a picture of Oprah and Beyoncé. There was a beautifully decorated home, the words "Big Deal," "Thankful," "Expand," "Grow," "Romance," and "Elvis Birthday 6/10." A photo of the Eiffel Tower that I had added to represent Anna, a picture of a ski slope, the words "Los Angeles."

The next day when I went to the hospital, I took Nick's board with me. I placed it right in his little window, in his sight line. He was undergoing a transformation, but he was rebuilding. It had been his vision at the beginning of the year. And just like he had described RuPaul with a simple "Because she's amazing," I knew the whole world would use those very same words when they talked about him.

That night, I saw a message telling me to look up the words to the song "Don't Give Up on Me" by Andy Grammer. I looked up the video, in which Grammer sings the song with a bunch of schoolkids. It was so emotional, and the lyrics were beautiful. It felt like he had written it specifically for us. It reminded me not to give up that night, and I listened to the words as tears streamed down my face. *"I will fight / I will fight for you . . ."*

I believed he would survive this with all of my heart, no matter how impossible it seemed.

eighteen

It had been eighty-five days since Nick was admitted into the ICU. I still sang "Live Your Life" every day, and every day people were still there, singing with me. It was astounding to see people from all over the world still so dedicated to our story. But they weren't just singing—mail was arriving at the hospital like letters to Santa at Christmas. There were piles of it every day, and I read to Nick each handwritten note and card. After so many days, I would have thought people would have stopped caring, but people just got more invested, more supportive, and more involved as time went on. Even with life slowly starting to normalize, they still had my back.

The world had begun to reopen, slowly, which felt strange. To see some people's lives returning to normal felt unfair. It was easier to handle how strange my life had become when I knew everyone else's was weird, too. I found myself annoyed at people I passed dining outside while I drove to and from the hospital. *They should be at home*, I thought. *Don't they understand what this virus can do?* I would drive by families walking on the street, fathers strolling or holding their babies. I was envious of them. *Why did he get to live? Why are they okay, but my husband is so sick?*

I would cry to my parents and ask, "Why isn't God answering my prayers?" I questioned God but never lost faith. I just wanted progress, one piece of good news. I was praying so hard, and trying so hard, and had been for so long. Why couldn't just one positive thing happen for Nick to make us feel like we were on the right track? I wondered. I would cry, but then pick myself up and get back to singing, dancing, praying, and cheerleading. I had to keep going, even if I was running on fumes.

Rachel knew I was hitting a breaking point, and she came over one night to have a socially distanced glass of wine with Anna and check on me.

It had been a rough visit at the hospital since Nick had not been very awake, and Debra had popped her head into the room to check on me. As the hospital's social worker, she had the job of making sure that I was okay, and she was a very kind woman. But I had hit my limit with doctors, nurses, and other hospital staff looking at me like I was fragile, crazy, or unrealistic. When Rachel asked me how I was *actually* doing, I went on a bit of a tangent.

"Honestly? I am just sick of everyone there looking at me, and talking to me, like I am a sad, wet puppy," I shouted.

I stood up and started to act out today's scene as I began to rant.

"Today I'm in there, doing my thing, dancing and playing my music, and in tiptoes Debra! And then she said in this sad, hushed tone, as she frowned at me, 'Amanda . . . how are you doing?'

"I was in the middle of doing Nick's arm exercises with him while singing along with the Four Seasons. She sees me there—choosing positivity, choosing happiness, and she walks in and talks to me like I'm a broken little kid! So I flashed her a huge smile as I kept moving Nick's arm up and down, and said, 'I'm just *great*! We're just doing some exercises! Everything is good here!'

"Then she says, 'I'm sure that Father's Day was really hard for you . . . ,' while shaking her head slowly.

"So I said, 'Actually, Debra, we had a *fantastic* Father's Day! Nick's levels were great, and we celebrated my brother and dad as a family! I got steaks, my sister made a pie . . . It was *great*! *It's all great!*'"

I had finally lost it, and they were both there, as usual, to be what I needed at that moment: an audience, an ear, a confidant. In hindsight, I can see that my criticism of Debra was completely unfair. She was just doing her job the way she had been trained to do it. She had every right to be worried about me. She knew my Father's Day had not actually been great, and she was only trying to show me sympathy and concern. It just wasn't what I needed at that moment. When someone is hurting, or going through something challenging, we think we need to use a hushed tone and apologize. But what I learned going through this is that sometimes what people need more than sympathy is an acknowledgment that they're being strong.

There was a lot on my mind that night besides the hospital. I knew that Anna was going to be leaving at the end of the week to go back to France for a bit. When she arrived in the States in March, she had left Paris in such a rush that she had brought only one suitcase with her. All her belongings were still there in an apartment she was renting, and her lease was up in July. She had to go back and pack everything up. She decided she would say goodbye to France and return to LA to rejoin the quaranteam through the rest of the year, at least. She told me she wouldn't leave until Nick was out of the hospital and in rehab. I was so sad at the thought of her leaving; I didn't want her to go at all and gently tried to talk her out of it, but I understood that she actually needed to go. It felt like an okay time, since the most chaotic days seemed finally to be behind us. Our days were so routine, and I had a whole network of help in place now. June was another month of ups and downs for Nick, but the hills weren't as terrifying this time. He was mostly stable, and so we were, too. We couldn't do anything but visit and hope and pray that he would slowly improve enough for the team of doctors to consider the lung transplant.

Anna and I were able to launch Hooray For the last week before she left. When the big box of our first thirty T-shirts arrived, we looked at each other and said, "Have we really done this?"

We had dreamed of having a business together for years; we had come up with several ideas but had never acted on one before. We had no idea if it would work, but we loved them, and so much had been done for us at this point that we were excited about this way to give back. We decided to donate half of the proceeds from our first two shirts to the World Health Organization's COVID-Solidarity Response Fund. We hoped we could make enough sales to donate at least a thousand dollars.

There was no time or ability to create any real kind of marketing campaign for our new company. One day we tried to get as "ready" as possible, and we walked around outside the house taking pictures of the shirts in different outfits we created. We used Anna's tripod to get one together, and then we created a Hooray For Instagram account, on which we could share the photos. We wore them for the first time during a three p.m. Instagram Live and announced our new company afterward. We walked around the bedroom, modeling, styling, and describing them like we were on QVC.

In our first week, we sold over one thousand shirts. We were floored!

We have since been able to donate over $50,000 to the World Health Organization's COVID fund, and that number grows daily. We were so amazed we created more designs, one each month, for which we donate 50 percent of the proceeds to a different charity. So far we have made donations to the Make-A-Wish Foundation, Hope for New York, the Sundara Fund, I Am a Voter, the Actors Fund, and Dr. Susan Love Foundation for Breast Cancer Research, and as the months go by, that list keeps growing. We created Hooray For during the saddest time in our lives to spread hope, and it remains one of our silver linings.

With the hospital now letting in visitors, Anna asked if she could visit again before she left. It had been over a month since she had seen Nick, and she wanted to say goodbye. Only one visitor was allowed in Nick's room at a time, so one day she met me at the hospital toward the end of my shift, and I switched places with her and sat in the waiting room. Nick had been very alert all day. He had his eyes wide open and was tracking movements. I warned her before that he had lost a lot of weight since she last saw him. I didn't want her to be alarmed.

I thought about everything while I waited for her. It had been over a month now since we were together as the Patient Pep Squad, over two months since Anna had joined me here in LA. I couldn't wrap my head around the idea of her actually leaving and was scared of how I would feel when she did. I had been living in such an alternate universe since March but had adjusted to it. It was all made bearable by my family's presence, by having my best friend there to laugh with, and cry with; the sister who would talk to me and cheer me up no matter how bad the day had been. Anna's leaving was going to be the first dose of reality. Todd and Diana were planning to go back to San Francisco for a bit in a few weeks. I knew the quaranteam couldn't last like this forever, but I didn't know how I would survive without them.

After about an hour, Anna emerged from Nick's room, red-eyed but smiling.

"It was so nice to see him again, Mandy, and to hold his hand," she said. "I think he looks great today. I told him he did."

Her good mood boosted my spirits.

He had stayed alert the whole time she talked to him, so she showed him pictures from Joshua Tree, played him a Tom Petty album, and talked to him as if it were just a normal day back in Manhattan, when she would drop by our apartment to join us for dinner, or to cuddle Elvis.

"I told him I was so happy he was my brother, and that I going to Paris just to pack up my stuff, and then I was coming back to LA with the rest of the family to stay until he was out of here," Anna said. "I told him that we had done it—the dream of relocating the entire family to Los Angeles had happened."

I n 2009, Anna wrote an email to everyone in our family that became famous. She had just graduated and taken a little trip to visit each of us siblings in our respective cities, which at the time were Houston, San Francisco, and New York. When she got home to my parents' house in Ohio, she drafted an email titled "The Kloots Family Relocation Plan." It read:

Hello Family,

I have become very sad that my typical week does not include spending time with my niece, nephews, brother, and sisters. I am always sad that my typical week does not include running errands with mom and playing gin with dad.

Wouldn't it be wonderful if we could all meet up for family dinners once a week? If on your way home from work, you could swing by to read a bedtime story to Hudson and Oliver? Or on a free afternoon, you could meet Tre and Nina at the pool and catch Nina at the bottom of the water slide? We have a huge family that all loves each other, and we never get to be together. We have adorable little children that are getting bigger every day, and we don't get to see them growing up. Imagine not having to worry about if you can make it home for Christmas? Imagine not having to worry about travel expenses and time off to see each other.

This is an extraordinary time in our lives as a family, and we're not making the best of it. I know our careers, opinions, and dreams have led us to cities all over the country, but I can't think of any dream better than getting to see my family whenever I wanted without having to take time off work and board a plane. Which I why I have come up with Operation Family Relocation 2016: my plan for everyone to relocate to the same city within the next 5 years so that we can stop missing out and start making the most of our greatest blessing, each other.

After careful consideration, I have concluded that the state of California has a bounty of things to please everyone.

Her email went on to cover more points and included some pleading. It was a dream, but an impossible one. We had jobs, houses, and lives spread all over the country. We couldn't all plan our lives to be in California or anywhere. With no commitment from anyone, Anna mostly gave up on the idea, but she would still bring it up from time to time, trying to convince us.

Nick wasn't a member of our family when this email went out, but he rechampioned the idea hard when he learned about it. He already had his sights set on living in LA, but he knew I didn't want to be that far from my family. So if we all were there, he knew I would be happy.

"I'm with you, Anners!" he said. "Let's make this happen!"

Nick always told me that if Anna and I went, everyone else would come. He saw us as the unofficial bandleaders of the family.

Anna was thrilled finally to have someone invested in her campaign, but at the time he proposed it, it was too late. My parents had decided to retire to New York and just rented a place. She had her own sights set on Paris and was already applying for a visa. Ali's husband's job was in New York, and my sister Traci had a small business in Houston.

So it was just Nick and me who went west in the end, never imagining that everyone would follow.

★   ★   ★

"The Kloots family relocation plan is happening, sister," Anna said to me as we walked down the hallway of the Saperstein tower together for the last time.

"After all these years! I told Nick that he made it happen, not us. *He's* the bandleader now. I also promised I'd bring back vacuum-sealed cheese from France, so we can have an ultimate cheese board to celebrate when he gets out of here. Triple-crème Brie for days."

We had a going-away party for Anna that night at the house. I wanted to thank her for everything she had done, so I got her favorite strawberry cake from Sprinkles bakery. We had a Mexican fiesta for dinner since Mexican food is one of the few things you cannot find better in France. The whole family was sad—none of us ever liked to see one of us leave. At dinner we did what we love to do: play our "go around the table" game where we say nice things about the person next to us. Lesley told Anna she was glad she had been here; she could help Nick beautifully write his story one day. After dinner, we watched *La La Land*, one of Anna's favorite movies. My mom, Anna, and I cuddled on the couch in matching PJs like when we were little girls. No matter how old I get, there is nothing more comforting than having my head in my mom's lap.

The morning of her flight, Anna strapped Elvis into his carrier for a final stroll through Laurel Canyon. As she walked back onto the driveway, crying, it began to rain. I saw her and started sobbing right away, too, and we stood outside in the sudden downpour together, hugging tightly, with Elvis squished between us. We both knew we would see each other again soon, but no matter what happened, things would be different when we did. These two months had been unique—some of our worst and yet best memories—and her departure felt like the end of something profoundly special. She had been my buddy through all of this. As she packed the last of her things, Elvis walked around the bedroom, taking items out of her suitcase, then ultimately deciding to just crawl right in himself. It was clear he didn't want her to leave either.

I went into a mild depression that night, and for the next few days, as reality set in that my best friend was gone. As often happens, you don't fully realize everything someone is doing until they leave. Anna had been whatever I needed, whenever I needed it, every day for the last three months. She was my understudy when I had to step out of one of my roles, someone to whom I could vent when I was angry, and a shoulder to cry on when I needed to sob. She was beside me dancing when I went live and next to me singing at Nick's bed. She took care of Elvis and me and found ways to make me laugh every day. She distracted, supported, and helped me through everything, and with her gone, I felt an additional void in my heart. I didn't want to lose anyone else, but I knew that, slowly, people would have to leave. It was a reality check I probably needed but didn't want to take just yet.

Reality was also seeping in at the hospital.

One of the things that gave me hope was meeting with the physical therapy team. Nick was still unable to move any part of his body, and his muscles had atrophied. His muscles had to be stronger to qualify for a lung transplant, and as a trainer I was ready to help. They showed me how to move his arms and shoulder joints. They showed me how to work his left leg and left foot. I could even maneuver his amputated right leg by holding his stump and rotating it in his hip joint. I taught Lesley everything as well so that she could do the exercises with him during her visits.

Dr. Ng was still performing bronchial sweeps when necessary. Some days there were barely any secretions, which made us so hopeful, but then his numbers on the vent would start increasing, and the next sweep would be bad again. We just couldn't catch a break; nothing seemed to be working enough to break the cycle. I was still talking to Dr. Larry and Dr. John daily, and they were always checking in with Dr. Ng. Nobody was giving up. In fact, we all kept hoping that Nick would catch one tiny break, which would then lead to a bigger break. Anything is possible in the ICU, and I clung to that.

Nick had been on the sixth floor at Saperstein since testing negative for COVID in April, but now they wanted to move him to the eighth floor. The eighth floor was more for long-term patients. It was odd, leaving six. We had really grown to love the nurses and some of the doctors; I had spent so much time there that it felt like a second home. They told us that Nick would get the same care on this new floor and that it was a bit less chaotic there. I thought a change of scenery would be nice for him.

In the afternoon as I was sitting with Nick, a male nurse whom I had never seen before walked into the room.

"Are you Amanda?" he asked.

"Yes," I replied.

"I was the nurse on duty when Nick went on the ventilator," he said.

"Oh my gosh," I said.

He told me that he was so glad to finally have a chance to speak with me because he wanted me to know that, before going on the ventilator, Nick had talked about how much he loved Elvis and me. He said Nick had even shown him pictures of us and told him about our new home in Laurel Canyon.

"He was afraid to go on the ventilator. Before he went under, he asked me, 'Will I see my wife and child again?' I'm glad you're here with him, Amanda," he said.

I thanked him through my tears, and he left the room.

I knew my mission. I had to get Elvis into this hospital.

We continued to have weekly meetings with the doctors each

Monday; they were essential to staying on track. The meetings provided a dose of reality to start the week, not something we wanted,
necessarily, but we had to go through them. Lesley and I would go all
week and weekend feeling hopeful by number improvements or eye
movements, but those small things weren't enough for the doctors.

This meeting was to discuss Nick's blood pressure. Today was a
check-in on a two-week trial they had done to see if they could improve
it. They needed positive results to keep moving ahead. While Nick's
blood pressure wasn't worse, it wasn't better either, and Lesley and I
knew it.

All the usual suspects were at the table, and we talked again about
what Nick would have to do to get a lung transplant; it was now the
only thing that could save his life. There was concern that even if he did
survive a transplant, he might not be strong enough to activate his new
lungs. You have to be able to move your body so that the lungs begin
functioning properly. Unlike a heart, which will beat for minutes outside the body, lungs need to be activated.

"Nick can't move at all," Lesley said. "It would take him a year,
maybe, even to walk. A year from getting out of this hospital?"

Everyone confirmed her question with gentle nods up and down.

We all knew that Nick needed this transplant to live, but it had become clear that there was no way he could get one.

Dr. Ng ended the meeting by admitting that Nick wasn't looking
good but that no decision would be forced on us. The meeting adjourned,
and I asked if Lesley and I could have a minute alone with Dr. Ng. As
soon as everyone left, I broke down. I started crying so hard that I could
barely get my words out.

"If we get to the point where we know Nick isn't going to make it,
I need to get Elvis in here. You have to help me. Nick *has* to see his son
one last time. He has to. Please promise me that you will get him in

here. I don't care if it's only for ten minutes, Nick has to see Elvis, and Elvis has to see his dad one more time."

My mask was soaked through with snot and tears. Dr. Ng reached into his jacket and pulled out a fresh mask. He handed it to me, saying, "I thought you might need this." Then he promised, "Amanda, I will do everything I can if we need to get Elvis in here."

nineteen

As the week went on, the option of comfort care loomed over Lesley and me. But the thought of it was so painful, we couldn't even discuss it aloud. I begged and pleaded with God each day: *If you are going to take Nick, please don't make us make that choice.*

At five in the morning on July 4, I got a call from a doctor at the hospital. I was asleep, but the moment my phone rang, I shot up and my heart stopped. I knew that a phone call that early, especially from a doctor, was not a good sign. From the moment I answered, I could tell this was serious. The doctor's tone was grave.

"Amanda, your husband had a bad night. He is rapidly declining. He is now back on both blood pressure medications, and they are completely maxed out."

I was shocked. "He's on both?" I repeated. "But yesterday, he was just on one—Levo—and his numbers were going down."

"Yes, he's on both," he said. "Things are not looking good, and you should get to the hospital as soon as possible."

This was the fourth time I had received a version of this phone call, which made me almost not want to believe it. But this time was different—I could tell.

"I have to bring my son," I told him.

"I'm not sure they'll allow that," the doctor said.

"I've told Dr. Ng that if this happens again, if you're telling me it's Nick's last day, I'm bringing my son to say goodbye to his father."

I called Lesley, who had also become used to, and perhaps somewhat numb to, these phone calls. She said she would meet us there, and I rushed to change and get Elvis dressed.

My dad drove us to the hospital, and I called Dr. Ng on the way there to let him know what the hospital had told me and that I was bringing Elvis. Again, I begged for his help to get Elvis inside. He told me he would do everything he could to help and would be there soon.

But when I arrived, nothing had been cleared.

"You're on the list—Elvis is not," the person at reception said.

"I'm not going upstairs without my son," I said.

"We're so sorry, but until we get a call clearing him, we cannot let him upstairs. You need to wait here."

My dad was outside the hospital, ready to help if necessary, as I begged the person at reception to let us upstairs. I was a nervous wreck, so when they said it would be at least fifteen minutes until this got resolved, I gave Elvis to my dad and went upstairs to be with Nick.

The moment I walked into his room, I could tell something had changed. The energy was different, and the row of machines on either side of his bed suddenly seemed to tower over his body. He was gray in color, and just lying there. The only sound was the ventilator, slowly helping him inhale and exhale. I put on music, took his hand, and waited for news.

Lesley arrived, and we finally got approval for Elvis to come upstairs, just for ten minutes. So I went down to get him and to give Lesley some time alone with Nick. I was angry. I had asked the hospital so many times—when Nick was having a good day—if I could bring Elvis, just for ten minutes, just so that Nick could see him and know that Elvis was there. Now that Elvis was finally allowed inside, it was too late. Elvis was here, but Nick was almost gone.

Nonetheless, I knew this was our last moment as a family, so I walked into his room holding Elvis and with a smile on my face, saying, "Nick, Elvis is here!"

Nick's eyes were mostly closed, so I felt like the only chance was of his hearing Elvis.

I spent our ten minutes tickling him and playing all his favorite games to try to make him laugh. Nick didn't react, but I believe he must have sensed his presence, or at least heard him giggle. The last thing I did was put our three hands together to have Lesley take a picture. There's a beautiful photo of Nick's, Matt's, Amanda's, and Lesley's hands stacked on top of Eduardo's before he passed away. I wanted the same for us. Then my dad took Elvis home, and Lesley and I spent the rest of the morning on either side of him, each holding a hand, with music playing. It was quiet on the floor, so we just sat there peacefully until a doctor came into the room.

Sarah was Dr. Ng's weekend substitute, so we had spent a lot of time with her already. She a wife and a mother, and we could relate to each other. She was incredibly kind, sweet, and empathetic, and she had become one of our favorite people at the hospital.

We stepped outside Nick's room with her, and she asked us how we were doing. There was no way to answer that question other than "terrible, devastated, and scared."

We told her that we didn't know what to do; we didn't want him to suffer. We didn't want to put him through additional pain.

She very calmly said to us, "I don't know if anyone has said these exact words to you, but hearing them may help you make this decision, in case he ever mentioned his wishes to you. Nick is now on one hundred percent life support, and he has been for a while. Every machine, every medication is at its maximum. That is all that is keeping him alive. His body isn't working anymore."

We had already had many talks about Nick's assistance and levels, but Sarah was right, no one had ever said those exact words.

Lesley and I had sat next to these machines every day, obsessing over the numbers and watching them take over his organs, but we had never thought of it in these terms. We had been in survival mode and hadn't been able to wrap our heads around losing the fight. What she said suddenly hit me like a ton of bricks.

Nick and I had never intentionally discussed this topic. Why would we? I'm thirty-eight, and he's forty-one. But strange things come up in passing sometimes, and he had actually said to me that he would never want to be kept alive by machines in a hospital bed. I had agreed.

After the doctor said that, I looked at Nick as though it was my first time walking into his room. He was less than half his size; his body was covered entirely with blankets to keep him warm. Only his thin, sunken face was showing. The dialysis machine was running his kidneys, a pacemaker was assisting his heart, he couldn't breathe without a ventilator, he had a trach down his throat and a feeding tube so he could "eat." The bedsore on his tailbone was getting worse by the day. He was covered in IVs, had been poked and prodded all over for months. He was missing his right leg, his left toes were black, and fingers of his right hand were black and swollen.

He was not Nick anymore.

There had been a time that he was. For a long time, he was there, and you could tell that he was fighting. But in these last couple of weeks, that had slowly changed. He was going, and I saw it that day. There wasn't anything left of him. Lesley and I both stood there, realizing all we could do now was be there to comfort him.

Lesley broke the silence, saying quietly, "Amanda, I think we're keeping him alive for us now."

"I think you're right, Mom," I replied, and we both began to cry.

When Dr. Ng arrived, he confirmed what we were feeling.

"I told you I would tell you if we got to the point where we were causing him more harm and pain than good," he said. "We're there now."

For the first time, we were all on the same page.

If he survived, the best-case scenario was that Nick would be on a ventilator for the rest of his life, a life he didn't want.

But we knew he would not survive. So now we could either choose comfort care, and ensure that he passed away surrounded by the people he loved, or we could keep going, causing all of us pain, and taking the chance that he would die in the middle of the night, alone.

We knew what we had to do but weren't ready to do it. We decided we would stay with him all day and sleep there so he wouldn't be alone in case he passed away. When night came, they didn't allow us both to be in the room, so I slept in a reclining chair next to Nick's bed, and Lesley offered to stay on a couch out in the waiting area.

I woke up at two a.m. and found the room empty of doctors and totally quiet. It had felt like such a grim place all day, but now, in the stillness of the night, it was strangely peaceful and almost beautiful. There was a dim, golden glow from the lights outside peeking through the blinds, and I got up and went to Nick's side. So much of this fight had been chaotic, but this moment was just calm.

I stood there, holding his hand and rubbing his head, and I said goodbye.

There was nothing new that I could say; I had said it all so many times now. But I knew this time was the last, and I knew that he could hear me.

"Nick, I have to tell you some things, okay? I love you so much, sweetheart. I will always love you. I promise you that I will do everything I can to be the best mom to Elvis. I will do everything for our little boy. I will give him the best life I can, and every chance in the world. I promise you that he will know who his dad was, and he will know your family—your sister and brother and your mom. I'll live in our house like you dreamed for us, and I'll try so hard to be happy for Elvis and for me. Thank you for our house, honey. I wish you could see it. You would love it so much.

"I hope you know the Lord, Nick; I hope he is with you right now. I pray you'll be our angel; please be our angel. Look over Elvis and me, and be with us.

"I will miss you every single day. We will all miss you every day. It's not fair that this happened to you; it's not fair that we have to lose you. I don't understand why this had to happen to you. I tried everything I could to save you. I hope you felt that. I'm so sorry I couldn't save you. Thank you for fighting so hard, Nick. I know you fought for so long to stay with us."

Then I rubbed his head as I cried and said over and over again:

"I love you. I love you. I love you.

"It's okay, it's okay, it's okay.

"I love you."

I later realized those were the exact words I said to Elvis when I first held him as he cried.

I said a big prayer over Nick, and I thanked God for everything we had together—our life, our love, our son, and when I was out of words, I softly put on "Our House," listening to it as I again sat down in the reclining chair and drifted back to sleep. "And rest your head for just five minutes / Everything is done."

It was the most beautiful gift—a perfect, peaceful moment alone with him.

When I woke up again, his room was busy with nurses tending to him and the machines. It was almost six a.m., and they were getting ready for the shift change. I stepped outside to check on Lesley and found her awake, too.

"Mom," I said through my tears, "I think it's time. We have to say goodbye."

We sat in the waiting room, holding hands and crying, talking it through together one last time. This is the worst decision a wife and mother could ever have to make, but we had to. I called Dr. Ng and I asked him to explain to us once more what happens when we choose comfort care. He told us how it would go, and explained that now that we had made this choice, my family could come to say goodbye and stay in the room with us. He would alert the nurses, who would start getting things ready. He would be there in half an hour.

Rachel came to stay with Elvis so that my parents and Todd could come to the hospital. While we waited, Lesley and I played music— Nick's music—and held his hands. I eventually put on a random '70s-themed station to have music playing for him.

The nurses told us he would probably pass away quickly once we started, so we waited for my family to get there and for Amanda and Matt to join us on FaceTime. My dad, mom, and Todd arrived. It was the first time they had been in the hospital, and though they had seen Nick in photos and videos, nothing could have really prepared them for the reality.

They walked in already in tears, but greeted Nick with love and told him he looked good. They each took a moment with Nick, and Dr. Ng appeared in the doorway, looking stoic. We all thanked him for everything he had done. For his empathy, and positivity, and friendship during the last ninety-five days. He was indeed an incredible doctor, and you could tell he cared for Nick, and for us, as he said a heartfelt apology for our loss.

They would start by giving Nick morphine so that he wouldn't feel any pain as he passed. I tried to keep calm, but as they began to administer it, I became hysterical.

I had known for weeks now that I was probably going to lose him;

we had made the choice to let him go, but the reality that the actual moment was upon us absolutely devastated me. There was no going back; I was going to lose him. I was crying so hard I couldn't see, or breathe, or stand. Without my family around me, I think I would have had a full-on panic attack. I kept apologizing to Nick, telling him I was so sorry as I sobbed through mask after mask.

When I caught my breath and got quiet, I noticed the song that was playing.

Nick and I used to debate who was the better DJ. I insisted it was me, with my Top 40 selections, and he insisted I was wrong. In our time together, he was always trying to teach me about music. Every day a new vinyl would show up at the door, and he would open it, put it on, and make me listen.

As the first machines were being turned off, I heard the chorus of the song that was playing repeating, "And I love you, yes, I love you . . ."

I asked my dad what song it was so I could remember.

"Nights in White Satin" by the Moody Blues.

I may have put on Spotify that day, but today Nick was the DJ, and it seemed as if he was using this song to tell me that he loved me one last time, over and over again.

We stood there as a family in a circle around Nick's bed, waiting, sobbing. We tried to calm ourselves as much as we could as the minutes ticked by. We had expected Nick to pass quickly, but his numbers were staying stable, despite his being disconnected from most of the machines.

I recognized the next song that came on: "Get Together" by the Youngbloods. "Some may come and some may go, he will surely pass."

This song is uplifting, and it made us smile even with what was happening. It seemed as if Nick was using this song to thank us for coming together through this and becoming one united family instead of two separate ones. He had always hoped for that—for all of us to know and love one another, and for us to keep one another comforted and happy. He would have wanted us to do our best to smile through this, and to keep smiling for him. We joined hands and started singing the chorus, *"Come on, people now, smile on your brother . . ."*

Nick couldn't speak, but at this point I fully believed he was talking to us through the music. The songs were too poetic, to perfect to be random. This song truly embodies who Nick was, his spirit, and what he believed in. It was him thanking us for coming together for him, and for one another. I didn't know how he was doing it, but I knew Nick was curating this music.

I wanted to tell them to stop so we could have more time, one more chance to save him. But instead, I watched as they took him off the last machine, the ventilator, and wheeled it away. Without it, he wouldn't be able to breathe. I knew these were his last minutes, so I looked over to see the name of the next song as it came on: "Going to California" by Led Zeppelin.

Nick was a huge Led Zeppelin fan; he had all of their albums on vinyl.

Up to this point, though, I had thought Led Zeppelin was a person and wouldn't have been able to name one song that "he" sang. Nick's face and lips turned white, and we watched him leave us as Led Zeppelin sang.

"Going to California" is an acoustic ballad that sounds like a grown-up's lullaby, a man tenderly singing about following his destiny to California to start a new life that awaits him there. I researched the song's meaning and lyrics later, wanting to understand what the song was about because it was so hauntingly beautiful. *"Made up my mind to make a new start, going to California with an aching in my heart."*

The song is known to have been inspired by Joni Mitchell. Nick pointed out Joni's house to me every time we went by it. The lyrics even mention "the canyons," and Robert Plant has said that the song reflects on "the days when things were really nice and simple, and everything was far out all the time."

Nick had wanted to come to California for that nice and simple life in Laurel Canyon.

The lyrics read like a monologue: Nick's last lines.

Toward the end of the song the tonality changes, and it sounds as if the words are actually coming from outside and above the vocalist's own body as he sings, "I think I might be sinking . . ."

Finally, the song ends with a reverb-drenched voice in the background, singing, "Ah, ah, ah, ah," as if the vocalist is falling away slowly, until the music fades out completely.

I had chills.

When you're on Broadway and suddenly find out that your show is closing, you feel this wave of sadness. As a cast member, there was nothing you could have done to save it. You didn't write the script; you didn't call the shots. You just had to show up, and smile, and dance, and perform, and give it your all every day. Your cast has become like your family, the theater like your home, and your dressing room like your own personal bedroom in that house, your space filled with photos, cards, and memories. After your last show, you have to take that all down, pack everything into a box, and walk out of the theater as it goes dark. I couldn't help but feel the analogy. Closing a show had happened to me too many times.

When *Bullets over Broadway* closed, I was devastated. The show had brought me so much joy, distraction, and confidence while dealing with my divorce. It was a stable paycheck for a job I enjoyed, and I had formed a family from that cast. It had also brought me Nick. The show closing just four months after it opened didn't feel fair. I felt as if I had lost everything I had just gained, and I was so worried about what would come next.

Nick, on the other hand, accepted it right away. He told me that when a show closed, he was sad, of course, but he also viewed it as a sign that it was time to move forward, to see what came next. He was the type of person who—once he had achieved something—ticked off that box and began thinking of the next dream. So while I cried as I packed up my dressing room and left the theater for the last time, Nick held his head high as he cleared his and walked out of the stage door ready for whatever came next.

I realized Nick's room had become my dressing room, the nurses and doctors my cast, and the hospital our theater. I slowly moved around Nick's room, taking down everything I had placed there over the last three months. There were cards and letters from people all over the world, poster-sized photos of us on the walls, three daily devotional books I had been reading, speakers to play him music, and his 2020 vision board. There was nothing else I could do now but put everything in a box and walk out as my theater went dark.

I passed Dr. Ng as I left and headed outside. I needed fresh air while I waited for Lesley and my family.

I felt so defeated. I had lost.

I had given this fight everything in me, but I had lost.

My mom told me later that she saw Dr. Ng, standing at his computer, his head in his hands, as I walked out for the last time.

twenty

The night after Nick passed away, Jono asked if he and the band could come to sing to us one last time. Lenii and Bill were leaving to go back to Ireland, and we were soon leaving to go to Ohio. I knew how difficult it would be, but I said yes.

My family and I headed out to the driveway as the truck drove up, still covered in twinkle lights. When I saw it, I thought of that first night they had come to play for us outside Brown Bear back in April. That night was the first time I had been told that Nick was not going to survive this. I had been told his lungs were too damaged, and he could never live like that. It was just Todd, Anna, and me then, at the very start of this. We huddled together on the steps of the cabin as we listened, and cried, and tried to process that we were going to lose him. It had been only three months ago, but it felt like a lifetime.

Molly and Trevor jumped out of the back of the truck once it stopped.

"Look who's with us," Molly said, holding out her phone. She had Anna on FaceTime. It was four in the morning in France, but Anna had stayed awake to be there.

"Hi, Kloots family," Jono said. "We came to sing you a song."

Bill started on the keyboard as Lenii began to sing.

This hurts like hell, but it feels right . . .

I'd heard this song every day at three p.m., and then a thousand other times throughout the last three months. It was the anthem of our fight. Earlier that day, I had gone live at three to sing "Live Your Life" with everyone one last time, and to say thank you to all of them. My eyes were so red and puffy, I had to wear sunglasses while I sang. I put on a pair of Nick's that he had bought at the Canyon Country Store, along with one of the flannels from his closet. Twenty thousand people joined me that day to say goodbye. I felt as if Nick was there with us for the first time, and singing the words out loud once more with everyone was cathartic.

Hearing it always inspired hope in me; it kept me going and captured the attention of hundreds of thousands of people all over the world. But hearing it that night, sung so beautifully and slowly, from a twinkle-lit pickup truck in the hills of Laurel Canyon, brought me closure. Nick's memory would always be alive here.

My family, my quaranteam, sat together on the driveway and listened. These "quarantine versions" of everyone in my family are forever burned in my mind now. I can close my eyes and see everyone in perfect detail: from the outfits they always wore, to their grown-out haircuts, to the expressions on their faces throughout the last month of this fight. No family ever imagines they will go through something like this, and no family is prepared for it when it happens. But my family had come together to take care of me in the most beautiful, natural way. We fought every day for Nick, but we also fought for one another, fought for hope, fought for love, and fought for life. Our bond as a family was stronger now than ever before. I saw that as the greatest silver lining, and I always will.

I sat there listening to Lenii sing with my arm linked with my mom's and my head on my dad's shoulder. It felt like the end of a sad movie, where the story didn't end the way you thought it would, but the final scene suits the storyline perfectly.

And it's all right, live your life.
Like you've got one night, live your life.
Yes, it's all right, live your life.
Like you've got one night, live your life.
They'll give you hell—but don't you let them kill your light, not with-
    out a fight.
Live your life.

The days after Nick died are foggy. I wasn't in denial, but it just
didn't feel like he was gone. It seemed like just another time that I
wasn't allowed to visit the hospital for a few days. It would take a bit of
time before the pain set in, and then the grief. It's still setting in, months
later. All I really felt at first were just defeat and overwhelming sadness.

I wouldn't have survived the week without my family. My mom and
Lesley helped me with Elvis, and my dad and Todd each set up a desk
in the office and took over the hundreds of phone calls. They worked
tirelessly as I wandered around the house in a daze, trying my best to
be a mom. This fight had consumed every moment, thought, and ounce
of energy for the last three months, and now, suddenly, it was over. No
more nights frantically doing Google searches, no more singing at three
p.m., no more mornings or afternoons spent next to Nick's hospital bed,
no more pep talks, no more phone calls with Dr. John, Dr. Larry, and
Dr. Ng. These people had entered my life and become the generals of my
army. It was so strange to realize I would no longer talk to them several
times a day. It was a huge adjustment for me. The battle was over, and
we had lost.

It had been three months since I didn't wake up and call the hospital
first thing for an update, three months since I had spent a full day with
Elvis without the worries of the hospital weighing on my mind. I felt,
yet again, how similar this was to the aftermath of closing a Broadway

show. There's a strange period actors go through as they realize, *I don't have to go to the theater anymore. I don't have to sing that song anymore. I don't have to do that dance ever again.* They almost don't know what to do with themselves, without the routine they've become so accustomed to; they forget what they used to do every day before that show opened, and they struggle to find their way to a new routine.

Everyone else in my life, everyone else in the world, knew what had happened, but Elvis was just a year old. Nothing had changed in his world, and he kept all of us laughing during the day as we tried to go through the motions. As Lesley had predicted, he was my reason to get out of bed and smile. But once he went to bed, the house got quiet, and reality began to sink in. I cried myself to sleep each night. That daily routine continued for a few days, and broke when Lesley decided to leave.

She had been away from home for six weeks and needed to get back to her other two children, the rest of her family, her friends. The Corderos were no strangers to loss, but how could any woman deal with suddenly losing her son just three years after suddenly losing her husband? She told me she wanted to spend as much time as she could with Elvis and my family before leaving, and so she spent every day with us. She took Elvis swimming, and we had long talks and family dinners. It was as close to normal as possible.

At night, we sorted through a big box of Nick's old photos and shared the stories behind them. We had a beautiful last few days together, and as she prepared to leave, I realized the bond my whole family had formed with her was another dream of Nick's that had been fulfilled. He loved my family, and he always told me, especially after his dad died, that he hoped his mom and I could become very close, but also that he really wanted her to get to know all of us.

Throughout this fight, I felt there was no way someone could survive so much and then not make it in the end. It didn't seem possible. And when I lost Nick, I questioned it further. He almost died so many times; if God was always going to take him, why did he draw it out so long?

But as a friend of mine pointed out, if Nick had died in April, no one would have known this story. I would have never started singing "Live Your Life"; I wouldn't have had the army of support and my family here to help. If Nick had died in May, Lesley, Matt, and Amanda would never have made it to LA. They wouldn't have been able to say goodbye. Lesley wouldn't have stayed, wouldn't have had the time with Elvis and my parents, wouldn't have become a real part of my family. If Nick had died in June, our house wouldn't have been finished. Elvis and I wouldn't have had anywhere to go and wouldn't have known if we could or should stay in LA. Anna would never have gone back to Paris and started living her own life.

It was a crazy revelation. It was as though he fought so hard each day and survived every near-death call so that we would all have time to take our places; then, once he knew everyone was taken care of, only then was it time for him to leave us. It sounded crazy, but it also sounded exactly like Nick.

My parents and I were going to leave soon, too, to go back to Ohio for a few weeks. So one evening, I came outside to look at the beautiful view of Los Angeles while it was still my backyard. I thought of Nick saying, "We just have to get to California . . . I smell opportunity in California."

Nick had wanted to move to LA so badly. He fought hard to get us here. He wanted a home in Laurel Canyon, and he wanted people to know and sing his music. He wanted to be a dad. It helped me know that he died with all of his dreams a reality, but it hurt so much that he couldn't be here to see it all happen.

I took out my phone and wrote a text message to Dr. Ng. I wanted to thank him for helping Nick and being so positive and so kind. "There aren't many doctors like you," I wrote. "I know Nick would have loved you. I wish you could have known him. I wish he would have been awake enough that you could have fought together, and become friends, and won. If you ever need someone to research anything," I wrote, "I'm your girl."

It was a light note on which to end a heavy message. Dr. Ng was always amazed by my numerous findings and ideas—whether they were possible for us to pursue or not. He always asked how and where I was getting all this information, and so quickly. John and Larry always told me if I wanted a career in medical research when this was all over, I could have it.

I knew the line would give him a laugh, and I figured he could use one.

I pressed send, and two seconds later, my phone rang.

"Dr. Ng! You already need something?" I joked.

"Amanda, how are you?" he said. "I've been thinking of you. I didn't know when it would be okay to call, but I've been wanting to check on you and talk to you. In the last three months, I've talked to you more than my own wife!"

Answering *how are you?* during a time of grieving is an impossible task. It would take a thousand words to describe how you actually are, and most of those words you can't even find when you try to. So you settle on *I'm okay* or *I'm doing the best I can*. But Dr. Ng and I had been through so much together, I knew I could be open and honest in answering that question, and I told him how defeated I felt and how sad I was.

He told me that this week he and the other doctors had sat down and looked at everything one last time. They looked to see if they would have, or could have, done anything differently.

"I don't think we made any mistakes," he said. "We really did all that we could for him."

I agreed, and I wanted him to know that I had always trusted him, and I thought that everything we did was exactly what we thought we were supposed to do at that time.

He told me he really appreciated that, and then he thanked me.

"As doctors, we have to deal with the patients, and all those emotions and complications, and then we have to deal with the families—which is sometimes even more difficult. You were a pleasure to go through this with, Amanda, and you handled this all in a way that I've never seen anyone do before in all my years of practicing medicine. Everyone here thought so."

My eyes filled with tears; it meant so much to me to hear him say that. I so often felt like the doctors and hospital staff thought I was crazy and delusional. I never knew if I was doing the right things for Nick. I knew my methods were unconventional, but I didn't know any other way. Keeping a positive outlook was for Elvis and for myself as much as it was for Nick. I was glad to know that it had helped the doctors and nurses, too.

"I'm quite a private person," Dr. Ng said. "I'm not on Instagram."

I laughed and confessed that I knew that already. I had looked for him.

"But I heard that you said many very nice things about me, and I can't tell you the number of people who have reached out to me because of that. That means a lot to me."

"I will forever and always sing your praises, Dr. Ng," I told him.

"I'm going to check up on you if that's okay," he said. "I'm going to give you a call here and there, and if you are ever sick, you call me. You have my cell phone number; not many people do."

I assured him that I would. And I told him one last time how much I had wanted that moment of walking out of the hospital together, how much I had believed it would happen, and how grateful I was to him that he had done everything he could.

"Thank you for being my positive doctor," I said.

"You know, Amanda"—he laughed—"I'm not usually that positive, that optimistic. That was because of you. You set the tone as positive from day one, and as a doctor, I think you adapt your attitude to the family and their outlook. You made me positive. Thank you for that."

The call was therapy that I needed more than I knew. Dr. Ng had become a key person in my life. I had been through more with him in the last three months than I had with anyone. It brought me peace to hear all of this from him, and it made me happy that, despite having endured this great tragedy together, we could talk and laugh like friends.

I had texted him because I wanted to thank him, but I never expected him to thank me in return. Lastly, he told me how serious COVID was still, how nervous he was even to be at the hospital. How worried he was for our country and the world. People weren't taking it seriously, and how sad that some people still didn't even believe it was real. He thanked me for bringing awareness to the reality of the damage it can do, to how dangerous it can be.

"People need to know, Amanda, and you helped to show them," he said.

When your life and your family are hit this hard by COVID, it's impossible to imagine that anyone does not understand that already, but in the weeks after Nick's death, I watched the numbers continue to climb as people refused to wear masks, as they began living normal lives again—like the virus wasn't a threat anymore. My life, my son's life, our family's lives will never return to normal.

Shortly after this call, we talked again, and Dr. Ng offered to be my primary doctor, promising to give me the best care possible. I knew it could be a bit difficult to see him regularly. It could trigger PTSD to be back in a room with him. I think some people would never want to see the hospital or the doctors again after losing a loved one. But I saw more beauty in the offer than fear. I trusted, respected, and loved Dr. Ng, and he had been such a confidant through all of this. I wanted to keep that connection, and I knew there was no one I would ever trust more with my life.

twenty-one

Our house is a very, very, very fine house on Love Street.

Leading up to moving in, I was preparing myself for feeling sad, scared, and lonely here. I wasn't sure I still wanted to live here, or even if I could. I knew all summer that when I moved in, it would mean that my family would all be gone, and I would be alone in the house Nick and I were supposed to live in together. But I promised Nick that Elvis and I would live here in the house he'd found for us, and be happy. I was surprised that once we moved in, my fears dissolved, and it felt strangely peaceful. It felt like my home, like our home.

Thanks to the GoFundMe, the rooms we'd hoped to slowly fix up over time were already transformed completely. Our contractor had been in the middle of the small renovation we had planned when we got the news that Nick's leg would have to be amputated. Within a few days, we had to scratch everything and make the house ADA accessible. We completely gutted the bathroom, ripping out the tub and replacing it with a walk-in shower. We enlarged all the doorways to make them wide enough for a wheelchair and ripped up the kitchen entirely to open it up to the living room, so it also presented no challenges for a wheelchair. The downstairs of the house, which we didn't have the money to renovate initially, we also gutted. We transformed it into a guest suite so that Lesley would be able to live there while Nick was in rehab, and now it works perfectly when family comes to visit and help me, which is often.

It's hard to believe sometimes that it is the same house Nick and I bought together. I wish he could see it now and enjoy it. He would be so proud of how it turned out.

My friend Michelle, my contractor, Bill, and Todd made all the decisions for me and created a beautiful home. In August, Todd helped me move everything in, hang pictures, buy plants, and settle in. He even suggested I "Canyonize" my front door. Many homes in the Canyon are a bit eccentric on the outside, paying tribute to the vibes here. I enlisted Molly's help; she is the unofficial mayor, after all, and a graphic designer. She came up with the plan to paint my front door with bold stripes of red, orange, yellow, and blue, like a rainbow, and I loved it. My addition to her vision was to write "Our House" above the doorway in bold, black letters. I smile every time I walk in the door.

It's bright, calming, and happy inside. The walls and decor are mostly white and soft gray, and when the sun comes up, light fills the living room and kitchen. It's a small home, but there's just enough room for Elvis and me. There's a big, comfy sofa in the center of the room, and a bookcase that holds a stack of coffee table books only Nick could have bought: Leonardo da Vinci, the Rolling Stones, Picasso, Prince, and Rauschenberg. Next to them are his record player and a hundred of his favorite vinyls that I kept from his collection. The others I gave to several of his closest friends and family members as I went through his things, knowing there was no better piece of him to share with the people he loved most. At the end of the bookcase is a lineup of toy trucks: Elvis's current obsession.

I received hundreds of gifts from my army after Nick's death, and among them was a painting of my favorite photo from our last photo shoot at Brown Bear. Nick is holding Elvis in his arms, and I'm standing next to him, smiling. The artist captured our faces so perfectly, it's almost impossible to believe it's a painting. I hung it on the wall of the living room, right next to the door. On the other side of the doorway is a giant, tie-dyed smiley face made just for Elvis and me by LA street artist Jimmy Paintz. It's my daily reminder to smile.

While I'm still not used to falling asleep alone, I have grown accustomed to waking up every morning with Elvis snuggled in my arms. He often wraps his little arms around my neck like he knows I need someone to hug me. Looking over at him in those first minutes of the morning helps me start each day with a grateful heart. He has gotten taller since the summer, but not heavier, so several pairs of his jammies from several months ago still fit him. He's wearing the ones with cookies and glasses of milk today.

We always have a few hours alone together in the morning before my day starts. "Shoes" is one of his only words, and it seems to be the first thing on his brain each day. This morning, he slides out of bed, grabs his tap shoes, and tries to put them on his feet while I film a Musical Morning, deciding to set it to "'Tain't Nobody's Biz-ness If I Do" from *Bullets over Broadway*. His tap shoes were a gift from Susan Stroman, the Broadway choreographer. She was so happy when Nick and I got married and then had Elvis. I play Nick's music all the time in the house and in the car, and Elvis has accepted it into his very limited playlist. He smiles when he hears Nick's voice and starts bobbing his head left to right.

"Oh, look who it is," I say to him, pointing toward the door with a big smile as Anna appears behind the screen.

"You're putting on a show already? You're only one year old, and it's only seven o'clock in the morning," she teases him, and then swoops him up for a big hug.

Anna came and surprised me the day before Thanksgiving. She self-quarantined for a month, secretly coordinated with my neighbors to sneak into the house while I was at tennis, shower, and be there to open the door holding Elvis when I got home. "I'm here for the next six weeks," she announced, and my heart, which had been heavy all day, suddenly felt lighter.

Prior to her arrival, I had spent the entire day driving around crying. Grief often takes you by surprise, and I'm learning strange things end up being difficult and triggering sadness. I've found that days before important holidays or important dates in our life together end up being extremely emotional for me. On the day of our wedding anniversary—and on Nick's birthday—I found myself so flooded with messages, calls, gifts, and love that the day passed quickly, and I didn't actually have time to think about the pain. But the day before those days is always quiet, and I spend it in fear of how I'll feel and what I'll do. I avoid the grocery store since that is also a place I have found it strangely difficult to be in. We always grocery shopped together, at the same store, and bought the same things. Some of those little moments that you would never think of as really mattering have haunted me most. As I go through the little motions of the day alone, instead of with my person, it hits me that he is gone.

As I go to make us my famous "gross coffee," I notice we're out of my creamer, so we decide to take a walk down to the Canyon Country Store to get another bottle.

"Oh, my best customer is here," Lily says to Elvis as we walk up. She has run the coffee shop outside the store for years.

"Hi, I'm Amanda's sister An—" Anna begins, but Lily interrupts her, saying, "Anna—I know. You live in Paris! You're here for the holidays? I'm so glad!"

Word that I wasn't alone anymore had spread fast. Elvis and I are a part of the neighborhood now; everyone knows us, knows my car, and now even knows my family members. I buy Elvis a croissant for his breakfast. It's one of the few things he genuinely loves to eat. He has one each weekend with his Stroller Buddy Eryn. She texts me every Saturday morning when she knows I have to teach a class at Bandier. But she never asks if I need help; instead, she writes, "Would Elvis like a walk this afternoon?" Like it's her privilege to come to get him. It's been eight months now that she has been walking him around the Canyon, playing him the Beach Boys. She has her standing date with Elvis while I teach a live workout class for my army, people all over the world who still want to sing and dance with me. I started doing this in August because I knew the weekends would be hard for me. I thought that if I could start my Saturday morning off with the energy of other people and a great workout, it would make me smile.

But today is Monday, and my workout is tennis. One of the first things I did to cope with my grief and the initial loneliness that set in after my family left was to pick up a new hobby. I had always wanted to learn how to play tennis, and I thought immersing myself in something new, and something that would keep me active, was important. Many of my friends already played, and I loved that it was a sport you could still practice during quarantine and into old age. I now take lessons twice a week, and sometimes I play with Aimee and Jacie, two of the women who started my GoFundMe back in March. We've become close friends, and it's a good feeling to have a new group of girlfriends in my life.

On the tennis court, I like that I don't have to think about the plan. It's nice to be taught after years of being the teacher. As a mom, and a business owner, it's nice to be bossed around by someone else for a change. For the drive home, I put on Nick's live concert at 54 Below. It's always comforting to hear his voice, and I often talk to him in the car, like he's there with me. Driving is another thing that I've found to be hard. I'm still new to living here, and all my best memories in LA are with Nick. As I pass restaurants where we ate or the places we loved, it triggers tears. I still can't drive past the hospital.

I call my mom and dad as I drive back to the house. I talk to them every morning and have a Sunday FaceTime ritual with the Corderos. It's so important that Elvis has a relationship with them, and these chats help me feel like Nick isn't gone. Elvis smiles big when he sees or hears his grandparents. He really knows who they are, and that's one of the greatest silver linings to this tragedy.

When I get back to the house, I can see Elvis and Anna through the patio's big window. She has him in his carrier still—she just got back from a walk around the Canyon.

"Aw, how was it?" I ask her.

"Well, I got a bit lost, my phone service died halfway into the walk, and my legs already ache from the hills," she says. "It's good to be back!"

I've only been inside for two minutes when my phone rings. I see it's my manager, so I go into my bedroom to take the call. For the last month, I had been testing for a morning television show on CBS called *The Talk*, which meant appearing on the show once or twice a week and seeing how I fit in with the other hosts and if the audience liked me. After years of auditioning for Broadway shows, this wasn't out of my wheelhouse. But instead of just having to impress the director, choreographer, and producer, this time, I had been auditioning for all of America. The show consists of five women from different backgrounds with different points of view, having discussions on current events, pop culture, contemporary issues, and family. Two of the hosts were leaving, and they were looking for replacements. It was a dream job, one that would change my life if I got it. My manager was calling to tell me about their decision.

Zach had told me, "Amanda, let me tell you a secret about Hollywood. If your manager and lawyer call together—you booked the job. If it's just your manager—you didn't."

When I answered the call, I realized my lawyer was on it, too, and my heart did a somersault. My lawyer calmly started talking, underplaying the news, "So, as of 2021, you're going to be officially joining *The Talk*..."

I ran out to the kitchen, where Anna was feeding Elvis lunch, and mouthed the words with tears in my eyes: *I got the job!*

Anna screamed, "OF COURSE YOU DID!"

This job will change my life; it's the first "real" job I've ever had. It will establish some much-needed routine in my day and provide me, for the first time, with a stable, reliable income and benefits. It is also in my comfort zone and feels like holding on to a little bit of my performing past. I have a dressing room to make home and decorate with posters, pictures, and little pieces of me. I'll put on "stage makeup" and a "costume" every morning. I'll do the show and then come home and have the rest of the day with my son.

Anna planned as much of a celebration as she could during California's second lockdown and COVID wave. We order a large pepperoni pizza; she got a nice bottle of wine and pints of ice cream from our favorite place, Salt & Straw. Elvis sits at the table with us in his high chair, and we all call out, "Cheers!" He lifts up his sippy cup full of milk and smiles like he knows how important this is.

"I wish I could have done more for you, Mandy. You deserve more of a celebration than this," Anna said. It reminded me of what Nick had said on my birthday.

"It's perfect, Annie," I tell her. "I'm just so happy you're here."

Being alone is hard. Being a single parent is harder. I feel the loss of my husband, my confidant, and Elvis's dad each and every day. My mornings and afternoons are busy and chaotic as I navigate my now four jobs. As a single mom, there is no built-in help. There is no one around whom you can quickly ask for help should you find yourself needing some. You must learn to plan it, and ask for it, and so I have. I have recognized I can't do this all alone and have become so thankful for the amazing group of friends and family around me, willing to jump in at the last minute, or come stay for weeks at a time.

There are days when I feel very strong and proud of what I'm doing, and days I let self-pity take over and complain to myself that this is not fair. I should have my husband, and Elvis should have his dad. It hurts when I realize Elvis won't know him and imagine the bond that they would have right now. I know Nick would have loved this stage, where Elvis is starting to talk and show his personality. He says "dada" so clearly, and it is the cutest yet saddest thing to hear. I think back on how badly Nick had wanted a daughter: his Ava. Having a boy had thrown us for a loop for a minute. But thank goodness we had Elvis; he is my mini Nick. He looks more like him every day, and he will carry on his name and his legacy. He will always be the most important man in my life, and I am thankful for that bond I know we'll have, and the one he has formed with his grandparents, uncles, aunties, and cousins. He's lucky to have so many people in his life who love and support him, as am I.

I still follow the same routine at night I always have with Elvis; there are just now some new additions. Since we replaced the bathtub with a shower for Nick, we don't have one, so I have to hose Elvis off with the shower instead of letting him soak and play in a bubble bath like most kids. I hose him off quickly as he stands there, crying. He absolutely hates it, and I tell him, "I'm sorry—I know this is not ideal, buddy, but this is what we have."

We brush his teeth, and pick out PJs, and then go into my bedroom, where there's a framed picture of Nick on my dresser. It's my favorite candid shot of him from our wedding day; he's in his tuxedo sitting in a chair in our first apartment together in New York.

"Let's say good night to dada," I say to Elvis.

"Dada," he repeats, taking the frame from me and kissing it.

Then we turn the lights out. I sing him "Our House" every night now, and then "La La Lu," and halfway through the song, he reaches for his crib. He lies on his belly, grabs a "lovey" in each hand, and pops his tiny bottom into the air as he closes his eyes.

It's so quiet in the house when Elvis goes to bed, and those final hours of the day are often the hardest. I usually turn the TV on so there's something to distract me, or FaceTime with someone while I eat. Then I watch something mindless and work on whatever I can until my eyes get too heavy to stay open anymore. I think about how, if Nick were here, we'd sit out on the patio under the bistro lights and share a nice bottle of wine, and then cook something together inside. His veggie gnocchi, probably. We'd put on a record and cuddle on the couch, and I'd fall asleep while he held me. I will always miss how that felt.

In a week, it will be December 5. It will have been five months since Nick died. In some ways, it gets easier as time passes after losing someone, but in other ways, it gets harder every day. I realize how much time has passed since I've been able to see him, hear his voice, hug him. I think about all he's missed and all he will continue to miss as more days, weeks, and months pass by. I want the time to pass, but I also don't, because I fear the memory of how he laughs, looks, and feels will fade as time goes on.

I want to keep the memory of him alive. I want to feel like even though he's gone, he isn't that far away.

I believe Nick is up in heaven watching over Elvis and me. I see signs from him all the time when I ask for them—rainbows in the sky, writings on walls, and, so often, songs on the radio. I have actually started to think God has put him in charge of curating the playlist for the rest of my life. But I also believe heaven isn't that far away.

A friend told me how when a baby is being created in the womb, it thinks it's alone because it can't see anyone. It doesn't know how close it is to its mother. It can hear and sense things and presences, but everything feels far away. But in reality, it's just a few inches away—the baby is right there with its mom—it just can't see that. But the mother knows.

The mother is carrying the baby the whole time and doing everything she can to care for and protect it.

Maybe when we lose someone, we become just like that growing baby. We think we are alone because we can't see anyone with us, but maybe the person we love is so close, carrying us, and doing everything they can to protect us.

I believe with all my heart that Nick is just a few inches away.

About a month ago, Elvis woke up next to me in bed at two a.m. He wasn't crying, fidgeting, or trying to breastfeed like he typically would at that hour. He was content, just staring up at the ceiling and making soft little coos. It was like he was in Fantasyland.

His noises woke me, but I lay there with my eyes closed, trying to pretend I was still asleep so he would drift off again. Despite my not making a sound, he just kept cooing, giggling, and making little movements, like he was interacting with someone. It was so out of character for him to behave like this in the middle of the night that I had to wonder, *Is Nick here?*

I had read that children are often visited by the spirits of loved ones because of their innocence and ability to believe in things that seem impossible once you're older.

So I lay there with my eyes closed and wondered if Nick wasn't here playing with Elvis right now. He was so content, I knew he had to be seeing something. I didn't want to make a sound, afraid it would disrupt Elvis's time in his own Fantasyland. So in my head, and to myself, I said, *Nick, if you're here with us . . . have Elvis give me a kiss.*

And just as I finished this thought, Elvis turned his tiny body toward me, grabbed my face, and pulled me into a long kiss.

Chills came over my body, and tears streamed down my face as his little lips touched mine. Elvis kept kissing me over and over again despite my not saying a word.

I lay there, sobbing, smiling.

epilogue

I imagined Nick's Code Rocky every day of this fight. As I sat next to him in the hospital, I'd paint the perfect picture for him of what it would be like.

"The whole world will be watching as you walk out of this hospital, honey," I said to him.

"Every doctor and nurse here will be there, lining the hallways, cheering you on and saying, 'That man defied the odds; we witnessed a miracle!' I will be right there by your side with Elvis, and your mom, and your family, and my family cheering you on. Every news outlet will be here, and people will be lining the streets outside this hospital. You are going to walk out of here, Nick. You have to believe that. You can do it. You are going to have a Code Rocky that inspires the whole world!"

Nick didn't get his Code Rocky. Sometimes I still can't believe that he didn't. I was so certain he would survive, so sure he would be able to tell the world *his* story. I felt the whole time that Nick was talking to God and learning something that he would eventually be able to share. He loved to learn, and loved to have deep, insightful conversations. I came to be at peace with the outcome, even though it wasn't what I wanted. I had to surrender to God's plan and try to find the lesson in it.

My brother, Todd, called me shortly after he got back to San

Francisco in September. It was his first weekend of real solitude since this all began, and he finally took some time to think and reflect. He told me that he had a revelation as he tried to "make sense out of something that made no sense."

My husband's fight and my family's struggle resonated with people all over the world.

We—Todd, Anna, and I—witnessed the innate kindness of humanity in a way we never had.

We witnessed that kindness extended to my whole family and to Nick's family as the weeks went on. We saw selflessness in a time when people should have been selfish. We experienced generosity in a time when everyone was struggling. We were overwhelmed with support in a time when no one had stability. We felt connection in a time of forced isolation.

A Code Rocky is the ultimate display of unity, and solitary, and love. It's a whole hospital uniting to rally behind someone, to cheer on a complete stranger. And Todd realized that although Nick did not get his, it's almost as if he gave us all a Code Rocky. He brought people together to witness and applaud, to cheer for the goodness of humanity at a time when we needed it most.

Nick was a people person—the last one to leave the party, the first to be there to help, someone everyone could rely on. He cared about the people in his life, and he always showed them kindess and love. His goodness radiated from him. Todd said, "It's because of his spirit, the way he touched so many people's lives, that people came to help the way that they did, and cared the way that they did. And now we will all strive to do that. This experience made us better people—kinder, more thoughtful people. You don't go through something like this without learning something, without changing,"

People have asked me how I stayed so strong and positive through this. In thinking about it, I have come to believe that it is during our hardest, most difficult times that our truest self is revealed. When the extras, and conveniences, and distractions of life are stripped away, we are also reduced to who we are at our core. From this experience, we witnessed firsthand that people are inherently good, kind, and caring. We also witnessed the impact of being that kind of person.

"Unfortunately," Todd said, "I didn't know Nick very well. But one of the biggest silver linings for me was that I got to see the best of humanity showing itself to you, and to us all—not only because of how you were processing this and remaining so positive, but because who Nick was as a person was being reflected back. I got to see aspects of his personality through the responses from other people saying how much he meant to them, and what an incredible man he was.

"It might be impossible to end this story on a positive note," he said, "but this is a way to try—to try to thank everyone for their love, support, and kindness that has forever left an imprint on our lives."

So I want to say thank you to everyone who was a part of this story, and who helped me tell it.

Nick sang "Live Your Life," with the lyrics as we now know them, only once live. It was at the encore to his one-man show at 54 Below in New York City in April 2019.

It's a common thing for Broadway actors who are out of work to put together a one-man show, where they sing several Broadway tunes and old standards. If it goes well, it's something you can then do in cities all over the country to make money. Nick decided to do one because he had been out of work for almost a year, and we had a new baby coming. He was starting to get worried and stressed that he would not be able to provide for Elvis the way he wanted to. So he decided to put together this show and record it so his managers would be able to use footage to get him bookings at other venues.

Looking back, it was the perfect blend of Nick's Broadway actor career with his "music band front man" past. But rather than just sing show tunes, Nick worked tirelessly on a set list that would give the audience insight into his life right now, and how he'd gotten there. I watched him for weeks as he pored over a hundred different pages of sheet music, worked on arrangements, and rehearsed diligently. I'd never seen him so stressed or devoted to anything at that point. He whittled one hundred songs down to two dozen: a mix of Broadway tunes and songs he loved from some of his favorite artists. When he told me he was going to sing "Live Your Life" as the encore, I honestly thought it was an odd choice. It was his original song, but no one knew it. An encore is usually something the artist knows will be a crowd-pleaser; it's something everyone can sing along with. It's supposed to bring the house down and keep everyone still humming for days later. But he was firm on ending with his original music, and making "Live Your Life" the encore.

I thought about the beauty in this choice as I listened to the recording when it was released on Nick's birthday, a few months after he died. An encore is an additional performance given by a performer after the planned show has ended, usually in response to extended applause from the audience. Nick wanted his encore to be "Live Your Life," and it was. It was his encore for ninety-five days while he fought in the ICU, and in response to the continuous, extended applause from his audience, it will remain his encore forever.

acknowledgments

It takes an army to write a book, and that is what I had.

Thank you to Lisa Sharkey for believing in me and this story before it was even finished. Thank you to my agent, Steve Troha, and editor, Matt Harper, for guiding us through the writing process.

Thank you to my family, especially Todd, Anna, and my mom and dad. To Lesley Cordero, Matt, and Amanda. Thank you to Dr. David Ng and the incredible doctors and nurses at Cedar Sinai Hospital. Thank you, Zach Braff, for giving us a home and thank you to the community in Laurel Canyon for the daily support.

Thank you, Hugh and Saskia Evans, for taking special care of Nick. Thank you to my 3pm army, who sang, danced, and prayed alongside me every day. Thank you to Elvis's stroller buddies. Thank you to Elvis for keeping me smiling every day.

To all the other doctors around the world who came to my aid.

author note

We wrote this book in six months, across two countries and time zones. It was challenging but important to us to share this story and relive everything that had happened, this time searching for meaning and metaphor within the tragedy. Our writing sessions often felt like therapy sessions as we remembered, grieved, and cried over phone calls and FaceTimes. With a nine-hour time difference, one of us would finish writing and go to bed just as the other was waking up and beginning the next chapter. We went back and forth for months, but finished the last chapter of this book together in Laurel Canyon as 2020 came to a close. We put Elvis to bed, opened a bottle of wine, and then sat side by side writing, sobbing.

As sisters we have always supported and believed in each other. We are so grateful to Lisa Sharkey, Matt Harper, and Steve Troha for believing in us, too, and supporting us through the writing process as first-time authors so graciously. One of us had always wanted to be an author; the other never imagined that she could. In writing together we were able to learn from each other, fill in missing gaps, recall stories and details from the past, and form connections to the future to make this book not just a recount of the ninety-five days Nick spent in the ICU, but what we hope is a tribute to his legacy, and many other things we value: the goodness of humanity, the importance of family, the power of faith, the joys of motherhood, and the unbreakable bond of sisterhood.

about the authors

AMANDA KLOOTS is a host on CBS's *The Talk* and a celebrity fitness trainer. After a decade of performing in several hit Broadway shows, national tours, and as a Radio City Rockette, Amanda started a company around her own unique fitness method and moved to Los Angeles with her late husband, Nick Cordero. During Nick's battle with COVID-19, her optimism and strength inspired people all over the world to pray, sing, and believe. Amanda currently lives in Laurel Canyon with their son, Elvis. They watch the trash trucks go by together Thursday morning, and always kiss Dada good night.

Together, Amanda and Anna Kloots created HOORAY FOR, an apparel company that celebrates the little joys in life and gives the proceeds back to various nonprofit organizations worldwide.

ANNA KLOOTS studied fashion in New York City, worked in interior design in London, and then traveled to 83 countries around the world writing and practicing photography before finally settling down in France and becoming what she always wanted to be—an author. Her essays are